I0783344

CARNIVORE DIET COOKBOOK FOR SENIORS

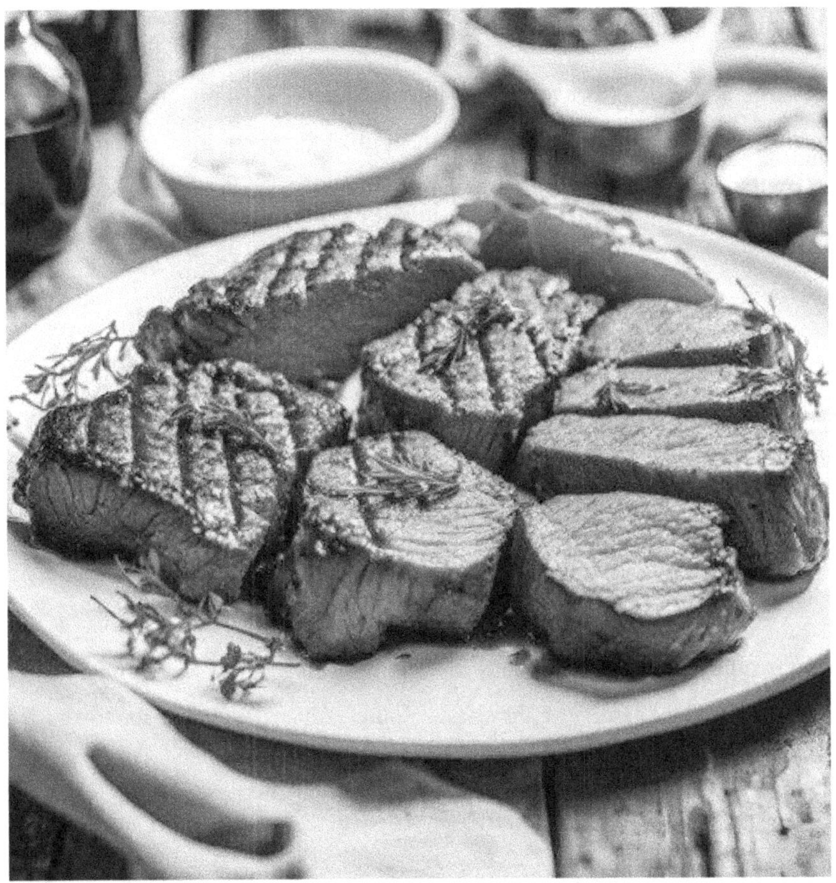

Patricia Grigsby

Copyright © 2024 by Patricia Grigsby

All rights reserved.

No part of this publication may be reproduced, stored in a retrieval system, or transmitted, in any form or by any means, electronic, mechanical, photocopying, recording or otherwise, without the prior written permission of the copyright holder.

This book is sold subject to the condition that it shall not, by way of trade or otherwise, be lent, re-sold, hired out or otherwise circulated without the publisher's prior consent in any form of binding or cover other than that in which it is published and without a similar condition including this condition being imposed on the subsequent purchaser.

The author has made every effort to ensure the accuracy and completeness of the Information contained in this book. However, the author and publisher assume no responsibility for errors, inaccuracies, omissions, or any inconsistency herein. Any slights of people, places or organizations are unintentional.

DISCLAIMER

The content within this book reflects my thoughts, experiences, and beliefs. It is meant for informational and entertainment purposes. While I have taken great care to provide accurate information, I cannot guarantee the absolute correctness or applicability of the content to every individual or situation. Please consult with relevant professionals for advice specific to your needs.

Contact the Author

Thank you for reading my book! I would love to hear from you, whether you have feedback, questions, or just want to share your thoughts. Your feedback means a lot to me and helps me improve as a writer.

Please don't hesitate to reach out to me through

contactpatriciagrigsby@gmail.com

I look forward to connecting with my readers and appreciate your support in this literary journey. Your thoughts and comments are valuable to me.

ABOUT THE AUTHOR

I am Patricia Grigsby, a passionate dietician with over two decades of experience in the field. My life has been a rollercoaster ride of challenges and triumphs, but through it all, my dedication to health and well-being has remained unwavering. Join me as I take you through my transformative journey, from battling health issues to embracing the carnivore diet and finding newfound vitality.

The Early Years Growing up, I always had a keen interest in health and nutrition. It wasn't just a career choice for me; it was a calling. As a young girl, I witnessed the impact of poor dietary habits on my own family members, and I vowed to make a difference. Little did I know that this determination would shape the course of my life.

The Roadblocks Despite my passion for nutrition, my journey was far from smooth sailing. I faced numerous health challenges that threatened to derail my ambitions. From chronic fatigue to digestive issues, each obstacle tested my resolve and pushed me to seek answers beyond conventional wisdom.

A Mother's Dilemma As a mother of three beautiful children—two boys and a girl—my health struggles took a toll on my ability to be present for them. Balancing motherhood with a demanding career seemed impossible at times, but my children became my driving force to overcome adversity and reclaim my vitality.

The Turning Point Frustrated by traditional dietary advice that offered little relief, I embarked on a journey of self-discovery. It was during this time that I stumbled upon the carnivore diet—a radical approach that challenged everything I thought I knew about nutrition. Sceptical yet desperate for change, I decided to take the plunge.

Embracing the Carnivore Lifestyle The carnivore diet was nothing short of a revelation for me. By eliminating plant-based foods and focusing solely on animal products, I experienced a dramatic improvement in my health and well-being. Gone were the days of fatigue and digestive distress; instead, I found newfound energy and mental clarity.

Advocating for Change Inspired by my own transformation, I made it my mission to share the benefits of the carnivore lifestyle with others. As a dietician, I understood the scepticism surrounding this unconventional approach, but I was determined to challenge the status quo and empower others to take control of their health.

Finding Balance While the carnivore diet has been a game-changer for me, I've learned the importance of balance and moderation in all aspects of life. As much as I advocate for animal-based nutrition, I recognize that it may not be suitable for everyone. My goal is to educate and support individuals on their unique health journeys, whatever path they choose to take.

A Legacy of Health and Wellness As I reflect on my journey, I am filled with gratitude for the challenges that have shaped me into the person I am today. My experiences have not only transformed my own life but have also inspired others to embrace change and prioritize their health. As I continue to advocate for holistic well-being, I am reminded that the greatest gift we can give ourselves is the gift of health.

<u>HOW TO THIS COOKBOOK</u>

Congratulations on choosing to explore the carnivore diet! Whether you're a seasoned practitioner or just starting out, a good cookbook can be your best ally in maintaining a satisfying and nutritious diet. Here's how to maximize the use of your carnivore diet cookbook:

1. **Familiarize Yourself with the Basics**: Before diving into recipes, take some time to understand the principles of the carnivore diet. Familiarize yourself with the foods you can eat and those to avoid. This will help you navigate through the cookbook more effectively.

2. **Browse Through the Recipes**: Take a quick look through all the recipes in the cookbook to get an idea of what's available. Pay attention to the variety of dishes offered, including main courses, sides, snacks, and desserts. This will help you plan your meals and ensure you have a diverse range of options.

3. **Note Any Special Instructions or Ingredients**: Some recipes may require specific ingredients or cooking techniques unique to the carnivore diet. Take note of these instructions and ensure you have everything you need before starting a recipe. This will save you time and frustration in the kitchen.

4. **Personalize Your Menu**: Once you're familiar with the recipes, create a meal plan that suits your preferences and dietary goals. Consider factors such as taste preferences, nutritional needs, and any dietary restrictions you may have. Don't be afraid to experiment with different combinations to keep your meals exciting.

5. **Plan Ahead**: Planning ahead is key to successfully following any diet, including the carnivore diet. Take some time each week to plan your meals,

make a shopping list, and prep ingredients in advance. This will help you stay organized and avoid last-minute decisions that could derail your progress.

6. **Experiment and Adapt**: While the cookbook provides a great starting point, don't be afraid to experiment with the recipes and adapt them to suit your taste and nutritional needs. Feel free to add or substitute ingredients as needed, keeping in mind the principles of the carnivore diet.

7. **Keep Track of Your Favorites**: As you try out different recipes, keep track of your Favorites for future reference. You can create a list of go-to meals that you enjoy and that fit well into your diet plan. This will make meal planning easier and ensure you always have delicious options on hand.

8. **Share Your Successes**: If you discover a particularly delicious recipe or come up with your own carnivore-friendly creation, don't hesitate to share it with others. Join online communities or forums dedicated to the carnivore diet, where you can exchange ideas, tips, and recipes with like-minded individuals.

9. **Stay Consistent and Flexible**: Finally, remember that consistency is key to seeing results on the carnivore diet. Stick to your meal plan as much as possible, but also be flexible and forgiving if you occasionally veer off track. Focus on progress rather than perfection, and enjoy the journey towards better health and well-being.

**** The Extra Special Bonuses are after Conclusion****

TABLE OF CONTENTS

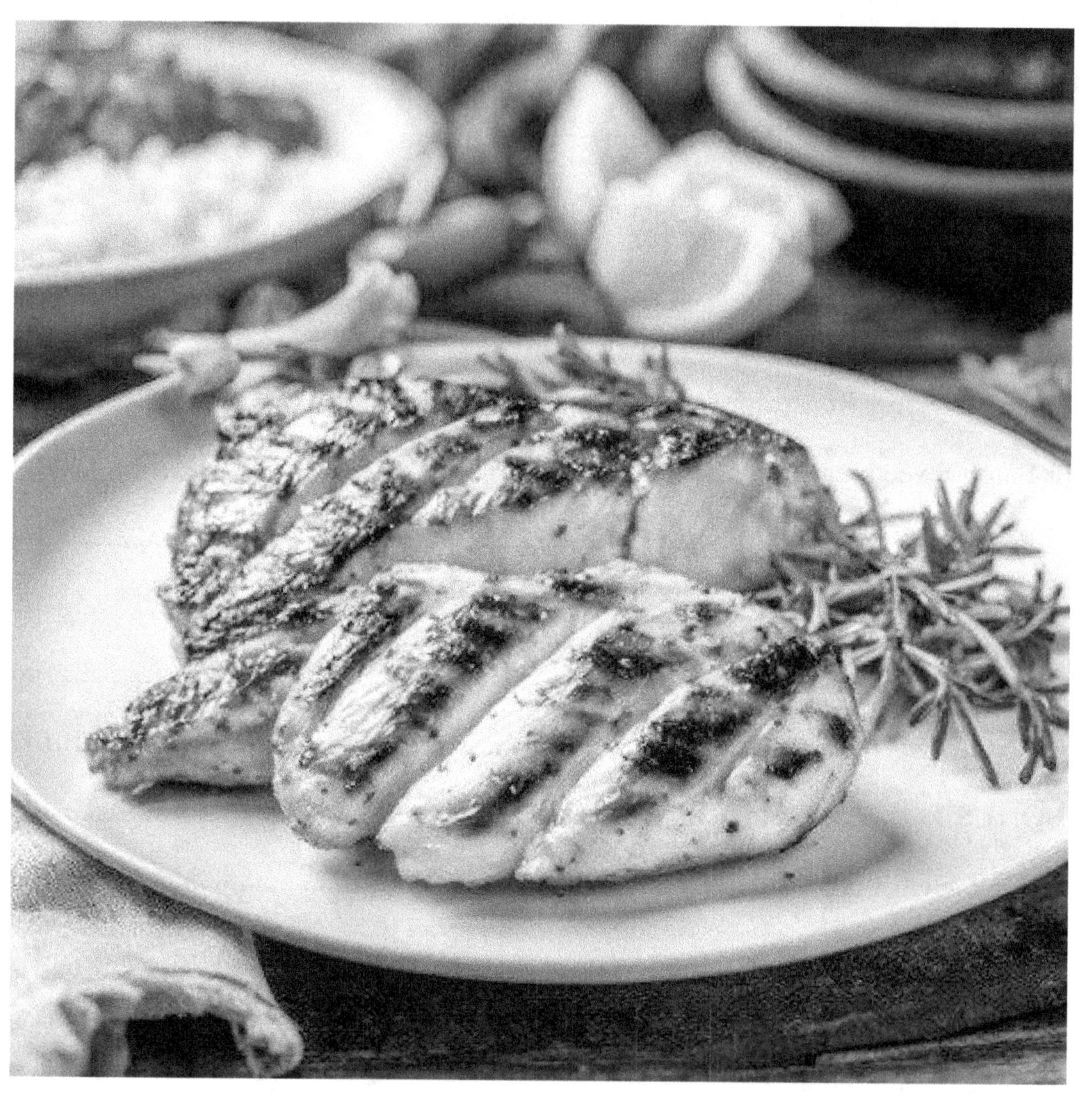

INTRODUCTION

Have you ever encountered a story that not only touched your heart but also ignited a spark of inspiration within your soul? For me, that transformative moment unfolded in the presence of Martha – a resilient senior whose journey resonated deeply within the chambers of my being.

Martha, a beacon of strength amidst life's tempests, her eyes reflecting a lifetime of triumphs and tribulations. As a devoted dietician, I've had the privilege of sharing nourishing meals with countless individuals, each harbouring their own hopes and fears. Yet, it was Martha's unwavering spirit that left an indelible imprint on my spirit.

Martha's path was one etched with resilience, each step a testament to her unyielding courage in the face of adversity. Battling chronic ailments and the relentless march of time, she found herself yearning for a lifeline – a glimmer of hope amidst the sea of medications and treatments. In her eyes, brimming with silent determination, I witnessed the profound impact that nutrition could wield over one's journey toward wellness.

Inspired by Martha's fortitude and unwavering resolve, I embarked on a quest to explore the transformative power of nutrition, particularly through the lens of the carnivore diet. What began as a professional pursuit soon blossomed into a deeply personal odyssey, a journey of self-discovery fuelled by the boundless potential of real, unprocessed foods.

In "Carnivore Diet Cookbook for Seniors," I extend an invitation to you, dear reader, to embark on your own voyage of self-discovery and empowerment. This cookbook transcends the realm of mere recipes; it serves as a testament to the resilience of the human spirit and the limitless potential for transformation, regardless of age or circumstance.

Within the pages of this book, you'll unearth a treasure trove of meticulously crafted recipes, each one a culinary masterpiece designed to cater to the unique nutritional needs of seniors. From succulent steaks to hearty stews, every dish is a symphony of Flavors, carefully composed to nourish both body and soul.

But " Carnivore Diet Cookbook for Seniors " is more than just a cookbook – it's a guiding light on the path to a vibrant and fulfilling life. By embracing the principles of the carnivore diet, you'll unlock a newfound sense of vitality, mental clarity, and overall well-being. Bid farewell to the constraints of conventional diets and embrace a lifestyle that celebrates the simplicity and purity of real, unadulterated foods.

So, as you immerse yourself in the pages of " Carnivore Diet Cookbook for Seniors," may you Savor every morsel, cherish every moment, and rediscover the joy of living life to the fullest. Let this cookbook be your steadfast companion on the journey to vitality, wellness, and, above all, the sheer ecstasy of embracing life's most precious moments.

Chapter 1
Understanding the Carnivore Diet

In recent years, the Carnivore Diet has gained significant attention as a unique approach to nutrition. Unlike many mainstream diets that emphasize variety and balance, the Carnivore Diet stands out for its simplicity and focus on animal-based foods. Advocates of this dietary approach believe that by exclusively consuming meat, fish, eggs, and certain animal products, they can achieve improved health, weight loss, and mental clarity.

The Carnivore Diet draws inspiration from the ancestral eating patterns of early humans, who primarily subsisted on meat and fish before the advent of agriculture. Proponents argue that our bodies are better adapted to metabolize animal foods efficiently, pointing to the high nutrient density of meat and its complete protein profile.

One of the primary principles of the Carnivore Diet is the exclusion of plant-based foods. This means abstaining from fruits, vegetables, grains, legumes, and other plant-derived foods. While this may seem counterintuitive to conventional nutritional wisdom, Carnivore Diet adherents claim that eliminating plant foods can alleviate digestive issues, reduce inflammation, and optimize overall health.

However, it's essential to acknowledge that the Carnivore Diet is highly controversial and lacks long-term scientific studies to support its efficacy and safety fully. Critics raise concerns about potential nutrient deficiencies, particularly in vitamins, minerals, and fiber, which are predominantly found in plant-based foods. Additionally, the long-term impacts on cardiovascular health, gut microbiota, and disease risk remain uncertain.

Despite the controversies, many individuals report subjective benefits from adopting the Carnivore Diet, including weight loss, increased energy levels, and improved mental clarity. Nevertheless, it's crucial for anyone considering this dietary approach to consult with a healthcare professional to ensure nutritional adequacy and monitor potential health risks.

History and Origins of the Carnivore Diet

The Carnivore Diet, although gaining popularity in recent years, has roots that stretch far back into human history. Its origins can be traced to the dietary patterns of our ancient ancestors and the evolutionary pressures they faced.

Early humans were hunter-gatherers, relying primarily on animal foods for sustenance. Before the advent of agriculture, our ancestors subsisted on a diet consisting mainly of meat, fish, and occasionally gathered plant foods. This lifestyle persisted for hundreds of thousands of years, shaping our physiology and metabolic pathways to efficiently process animal-based nutrients.

While the Carnivore Diet has historical precedents, its contemporary popularity can also be attributed to a growing dissatisfaction with conventional dietary advice and the rise of the "ancestral health" movement. Proponents argue that our bodies are better adapted to metabolize animal foods, citing evidence of improved markers of health and vitality among those who adhere to the diet.

Despite its ancient roots, the Carnivore Diet remains a topic of debate among nutritionists, scientists, and healthcare professionals. Skeptics raise concerns about potential nutrient deficiencies, the lack of long-term research, and the sustainability of a diet based solely on animal products. Critics also point to the diversity of traditional diets around the world, which often include plant foods, as evidence against the exclusivity of the Carnivore Diet.

Scientific Principles Behind the Carnivore Diet

The Carnivore Diet is based on several scientific principles, albeit controversial ones, that proponents argue support its efficacy and potential benefits for health and well-being.

1. **Evolutionary Biology:** Advocates of the Carnivore Diet point to our evolutionary history as evidence of our adaptation to consuming animal-based foods. They argue that for much of human evolution, our ancestors subsisted primarily on meat and fish, suggesting that our bodies are well-equipped to derive essential nutrients from animal sources.

2. **Nutrient Density:** Animal foods, such as meat, fish, and eggs, are highly nutrient-dense, containing essential vitamins, minerals, and amino acids necessary for optimal health. Proponents of the Carnivore Diet argue that by focusing exclusively on these nutrient-rich foods, individuals can meet their nutritional needs more efficiently compared to diets that include plant-based foods.

3. **Complete Protein Profile:** Meat is a complete source of protein, meaning it contains all nine essential amino acids that the body cannot produce on its own. This makes animal foods an excellent source of high-quality protein, which is crucial for muscle growth, tissue repair, and various metabolic processes.

4. **Elimination of Antinutrients:** Plant foods contain compounds known as antinutrients, such as lectins, phytates, and oxalates, which can interfere with nutrient absorption and cause digestive discomfort in some individuals. By excluding plant foods from the diet, proponents of the Carnivore Diet argue that they can alleviate digestive issues and improve nutrient absorption.

5. **Reduction of Inflammatory Foods:** Certain plant foods, particularly grains, legumes, and nightshade vegetables, contain compounds that may trigger inflammation in susceptible individuals. By eliminating these potentially inflammatory foods, the Carnivore Diet aims to reduce systemic inflammation and alleviate symptoms of conditions like autoimmune diseases and digestive disorders.

6. **Potential for Gut Healing:** Some proponents suggest that the Carnivore Diet may promote gut healing by removing common dietary irritants and allowing the digestive system to rest and repair. Additionally, the high protein content of animal foods may support the growth of beneficial gut bacteria and contribute to a healthier gut microbiome.

While these scientific principles form the basis of the Carnivore Diet, it's essential to acknowledge that the diet remains highly controversial within the scientific and medical communities. Critics raise concerns about potential nutrient deficiencies, the lack of long-term research, and the sustainability of a diet that excludes plant-based foods.

Benefits of the Carnivore Diet for Women Over 60

The Carnivore Diet, which primarily consists of animal products like meat, fish, and animal-derived fats, has garnered attention for its potential benefits across various demographics. For seniors, in particular, this diet may offer several advantages:

1. **Nutrient Density**: As people age, their bodies may become less efficient at absorbing nutrients. Animal products are dense sources of essential nutrients like protein, vitamins (such as B12 and D), and minerals (like iron and zinc), which are crucial for maintaining overall health, muscle mass, and cognitive function.

2. **Simplicity**: The Carnivore Diet is straightforward, eliminating the need for complicated meal planning or tracking of multiple food groups. For seniors who may face challenges with meal preparation or have reduced appetites, this simplicity can be advantageous.

3. **Reduced Inflammation**: Some proponents of the Carnivore Diet suggest that eliminating plant foods can reduce inflammation in the body, which is associated with various age-related conditions such as arthritis and cardiovascular disease. While more research is needed, anecdotal evidence suggests that some individuals experience decreased joint pain and improved mobility on this diet.

4. **Blood Sugar Regulation**: By excluding carbohydrates, the Carnivore Diet may help stabilize blood sugar levels, which is especially beneficial for seniors with diabetes or those at risk of developing insulin resistance.

5. **Weight Management**: Seniors often face challenges with maintaining a healthy weight due to changes in metabolism and decreased physical activity. The high protein content of the Carnivore Diet can help promote satiety and preserve muscle mass, which may support weight management goals.

6. **Improved Digestive Health**: For seniors with digestive issues such as irritable bowel syndrome (IBS) or inflammatory bowel disease (IBD), eliminating fiber-rich plant foods can alleviate symptoms and provide relief from gastrointestinal discomfort.

7. **Increased Energy**: Some seniors report feeling more energized and mentally sharp on the Carnivore Diet, possibly due to the stable blood sugar levels and elimination of foods that may cause fatigue or brain fog.

Despite these potential benefits, it's essential for seniors considering the Carnivore Diet to consult with a healthcare professional before making any significant dietary changes. Individual nutritional needs, existing health conditions, and medication interactions should all be taken into account to ensure that this diet is safe and appropriate. Additionally, seniors should prioritize consuming high-quality animal products, including lean meats and fatty fish, while staying hydrated and incorporating any necessary supplements to address potential nutrient deficiencies.

Debunking Common Myths and Misconceptions

The Carnivore Diet has sparked a range of opinions and misconceptions. Here, we debunk some of the most common myths surrounding this controversial dietary approach:

Myth 1: The Carnivore Diet is Unhealthy Due to the Lack of Nutrient Variety. Reality: While the Carnivore Diet is indeed restrictive, animal foods such as meat, fish, and eggs are highly nutritious and contain essential vitamins, minerals, and amino acids. With careful planning and supplementation, it's possible to meet most nutrient needs on this diet.

Myth 2: Plant Foods are Essential for Fiber Intake and Digestive Health. Reality: While fiber is important for digestive health, it is not essential for everyone, and some individuals may thrive without it. The Carnivore Diet may lead to changes in bowel habits, but many adherents report improvements in digestive issues such as bloating and gas.

Myth 3: The Carnivore Diet Causes Nutrient Deficiencies. Reality: While it's true that the Carnivore Diet lacks certain nutrients found in plant foods, such as vitamin C and fiber, deficiencies can be mitigated through careful food selection and supplementation. Many individuals on the Carnivore Diet undergo regular blood tests to monitor their nutrient levels and adjust their diet accordingly.

Myth 4: The Carnivore Diet Increases the Risk of Heart Disease. Reality: While the Carnivore Diet is high in saturated fat and cholesterol from animal foods, recent research suggests that these dietary components may not have as significant an impact on heart health as previously believed. However, long-term studies are needed to fully understand the diet's effects on cardiovascular health.

Myth 5: The Carnivore Diet is Unsustainable and Unethical. Reality: While the Carnivore Diet may not align with certain ethical and environmental beliefs, it's essential to recognize that dietary choices are highly individual. Some individuals may choose the Carnivore Diet for health reasons or due to specific dietary intolerances or preferences.

Myth 6: The Carnivore Diet is Only for Weight Loss. Reality: While weight loss is a common goal for many individuals on the Carnivore Diet, others adopt it for reasons such as improved mental clarity, energy levels, and overall health. The diet can be customized to meet various health and lifestyle goals.

while the Carnivore Diet may challenge conventional dietary norms and raise concerns among some health professionals, it's important to separate fact from fiction and consider the individual experiences and motivations behind dietary choices. Like any dietary approach, the Carnivore Diet has its potential benefits and limitations, and individuals should carefully weigh these factors.

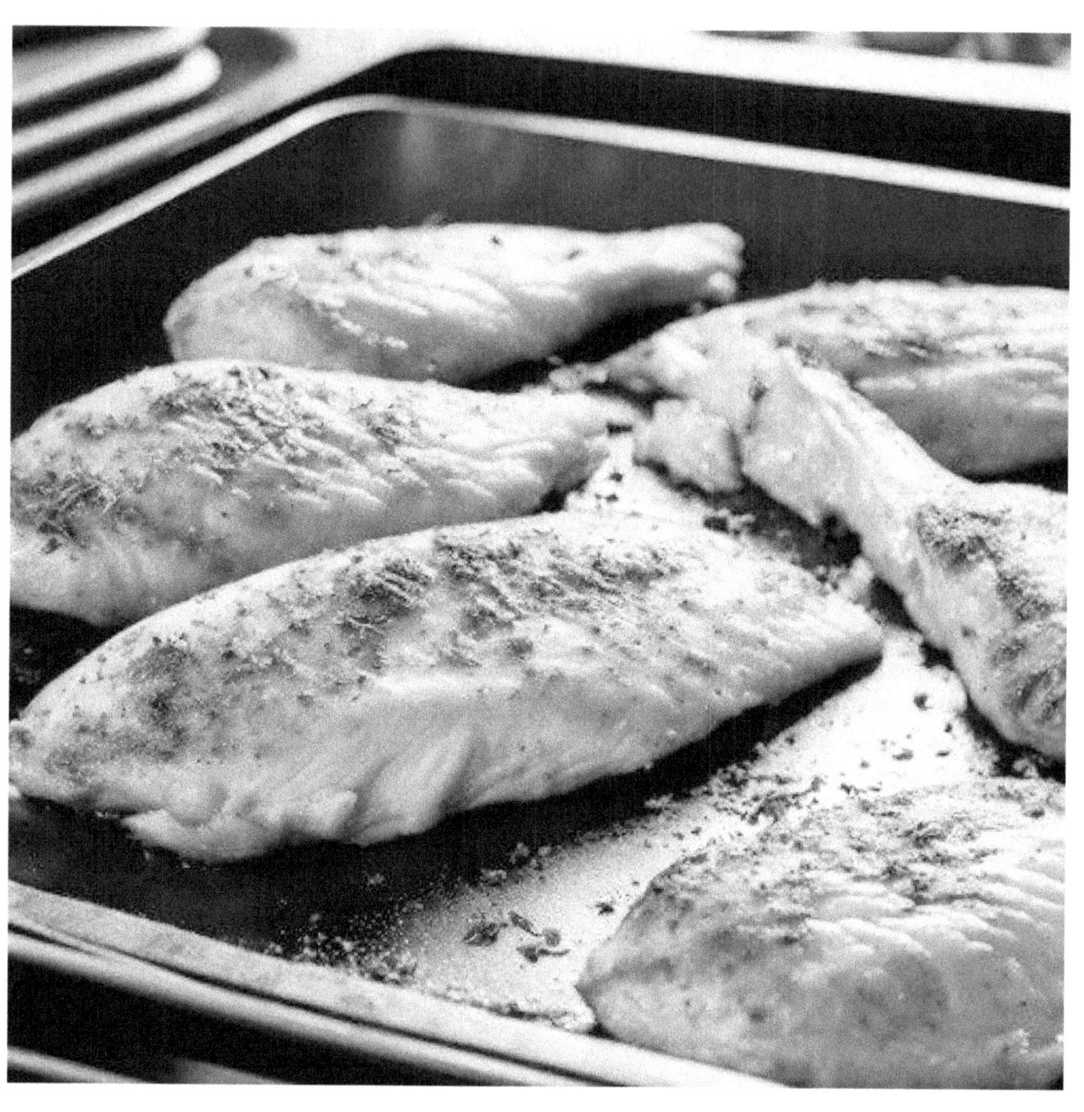

Chapter 2
Anatomy of the Carnivore Diet

The Carnivore Diet is a dietary approach that revolves around the consumption of animal-based foods while excluding plant-based foods. Here's a breakdown of the key components and principles that make up the anatomy of the Carnivore Diet:

1. **Animal-Based Foods**: The foundation of the Carnivore Diet consists of meat, fish, and poultry. These animal foods provide essential nutrients such as protein, fat, vitamins, and minerals necessary for optimal health. Organ meats, such as liver and kidney, are also encouraged for their high nutrient density.

2. **Eggs:** Eggs are a staple of the Carnivore Diet due to their nutrient-rich profile, including high-quality protein, vitamins, and minerals. They can be consumed in various forms, such as scrambled, boiled, or fried.

3. **Dairy (Optional):** Some individuals on the Carnivore Diet choose to include dairy products such as cheese, butter, and heavy cream. While dairy is not strictly necessary, it can provide additional sources of fat and nutrients for those who tolerate it well.

4. **Water:** Although not a food, water is a crucial component of the Carnivore Diet. Adequate hydration is essential for overall health and proper bodily function, especially when consuming a diet high in protein and fat.

5. **Salt:** Salt is often recommended on the Carnivore Diet to ensure adequate electrolyte balance, especially during the initial adaptation phase. Many Carnivore Diet practitioners prefer unrefined salts, such as sea salt or Himalayan salt, for their mineral content.

6. **Beverages:** While water is the primary beverage on the Carnivore Diet, some individuals may also include black coffee or herbal tea without added sweeteners or additives. These beverages can be consumed in moderation and are typically considered acceptable on the diet.

7. **Exclusion of Plant-Based Foods:** One of the defining features of the Carnivore Diet is the exclusion of plant-based foods such as fruits, vegetables, grains, legumes, nuts, seeds, and oils. This restriction is based on the belief that these foods may contribute to digestive issues, inflammation, and nutrient imbalances in some individuals.

8. **Processed Foods**: Processed foods, including refined carbohydrates, sugars, vegetable oils, and artificial additives, are strictly avoided on the Carnivore Diet. The focus is on whole, minimally processed animal-based foods to maximize nutrient intake and promote overall health.

9. **Personalization:** The Carnivore Diet can be personalized to individual preferences and goals. Some people may choose to include specific types of animal foods or variations of the diet, such as incorporating intermittent fasting or cycling between periods of strict carnivory and more flexible eating patterns.

Macronutrient Breakdown: Protein, Fat, and Minimal Carbohydrates

The Carnivore Diet is characterized by its specific macronutrient breakdown, primarily consisting of protein and fat while minimizing carbohydrate intake. Here's a closer look at the macronutrient composition of the Carnivore Diet:

1. **Protein:** Protein is a foundational component of the Carnivore Diet, providing the building blocks necessary for muscle growth, tissue repair, and various metabolic processes. Animal-based foods such as meat, fish, poultry, and eggs are rich sources of high-quality protein. The recommended protein intake on the Carnivore Diet typically ranges from moderate to high levels, depending on individual needs and activity levels.

2. **Fat:** Fat is another essential macronutrient on the Carnivore Diet, providing a concentrated source of energy and supporting various physiological functions. Animal foods naturally contain fats, including saturated fats, monounsaturated fats, and, in smaller amounts, polyunsaturated fats. Fatty cuts of meat, oily fish, and animal-derived fats like butter and tallow are common sources of dietary fat on the Carnivore Diet. Fat intake is often emphasized to ensure satiety, energy balance, and optimal nutrient absorption.

3. **Carbohydrates:** Carbohydrates are kept to a minimum on the Carnivore Diet, with the exclusion of most plant-based foods. While animal foods may contain trace amounts of carbohydrates, they are negligible compared to the carbohydrate content of plant foods. By minimizing carbohydrate intake, the Carnivore Diet aims to reduce blood sugar and insulin levels, promote fat metabolism for energy, and potentially alleviate symptoms of conditions such as insulin resistance and metabolic syndrome.

Overall, the macronutrient breakdown of the Carnivore Diet typically emphasizes high protein and fat intake while restricting carbohydrates to minimal levels. This dietary approach prioritizes nutrient-dense animal-based foods while excluding plant-based sources of carbohydrates, with the goal of optimizing metabolic health, promoting satiety, and supporting overall well-being. As with any dietary regimen, individual macronutrient needs may vary based on factors such as age, gender, activity level, and health status, and adjustments may be necessary to achieve optimal results on the Carnivore Diet

Nutritional Considerations and Micronutrient Sources

While the Carnivore Diet focuses primarily on animal-based foods, ensuring adequate intake of essential vitamins and minerals is crucial for maintaining overall health and well-being. Here are some nutritional considerations and key micronutrient sources to keep in mind when following the Carnivore Diet:

1. **Vitamin B12:** Vitamin B12 is primarily found in animal foods and is essential for red blood cell formation, neurological function, and DNA synthesis. Good sources of vitamin B12 on the Carnivore Diet include beef, liver, fish, shellfish, and eggs.

2. **Iron:** Iron is necessary for oxygen transport in the blood and plays a vital role in energy production and immune function. Animal foods such as red meat, organ meats (especially liver), and shellfish are rich sources of heme iron, which is more readily absorbed by the body compared to non-heme iron found in plant foods.

3. **Zinc:** Zinc is important for immune function, wound healing, and DNA synthesis. Animal foods such as red meat, shellfish, poultry, and eggs are excellent sources of zinc. Including a variety of these foods in the diet can help ensure adequate zinc intake.

4. **Vitamin D:** Vitamin D is essential for bone health, immune function, and overall well-being. While vitamin D is primarily obtained through sun exposure, some animal foods such as fatty fish (e.g., salmon, mackerel) and egg yolks also contain small amounts of vitamin D.

5. **Omega-3 Fatty Acids:** Omega-3 fatty acids are important for heart health, brain function, and reducing inflammation. Fatty fish such as salmon,

sardines, and mackerel are excellent sources of omega-3 fatty acids, particularly EPA and DHA.

6. **Electrolytes:** Maintaining electrolyte balance is essential for proper hydration, nerve function, and muscle contractions. Including sources of sodium, potassium, and magnesium in the diet can help prevent electrolyte imbalances. Salt, beef, pork, fish, and shellfish are good sources of sodium, while potassium can be found in meats, fish, and some dairy products. Magnesium-rich foods include nuts, seeds, and certain fish.

7. **Vitamin A:** Vitamin A is important for vision, immune function, and skin health. Animal foods such as liver, egg yolks, and fatty fish contain preformed vitamin A (retinol), while some plant foods provide beta-carotene, a precursor that the body can convert into vitamin A.

While animal-based foods provide many essential nutrients, individuals on the Carnivore Diet may still benefit from supplementation or strategic food choices to ensure optimal intake of certain vitamins and minerals.

Fasting and Intermittent Feeding in the Carnivore Diet

Fasting and intermittent feeding strategies are commonly incorporated into the Carnivore Diet by many practitioners to enhance its potential benefits and improve metabolic flexibility. Here's a closer look at how fasting and intermittent feeding can be integrated into the Carnivore Diet:

1. **Intermittent Fasting:** Intermittent fasting (IF) involves cycling between periods of eating and fasting, typically on a daily basis. Common IF protocols include the 16/8 method, where individuals fast for 16 hours and eat within an 8-hour window, and the 24-hour fast, where individuals consume one meal a day (OMAD) within a 24-hour period. On the Carnivore Diet, individuals may choose to practice intermittent fasting to promote fat metabolism, improve insulin sensitivity, and enhance overall metabolic health.

2. **Extended Fasting:** Extended fasting involves fasting for longer periods, typically ranging from 24 hours to several days. Some individuals on the Carnivore Diet may incorporate extended fasting as a way to accelerate fat loss, promote autophagy (cellular repair), and reset metabolic processes. Extended fasting should be approached cautiously and under the guidance of a healthcare professional, especially for those with underlying health conditions or nutrient deficiencies.

3. **Fat Adaptation:** Fasting and intermittent feeding can help promote fat adaptation, where the body becomes more efficient at utilizing fat for fuel in the absence of carbohydrates. On the Carnivore Diet, which is naturally low in carbohydrates, fat adaptation is a key metabolic adaptation that may

lead to increased energy levels, improved mental clarity, and better appetite control.

4. **Meal Timing and Frequency:** Some individuals on the Carnivore Diet may choose to eat two or three larger meals within their feeding window, while others may prefer smaller, more frequent meals. The optimal meal timing and frequency can vary based on individual preferences, lifestyle factors, and metabolic goals. Experimenting with different meal timing and frequency can help individuals find a pattern that works best for them while following the Carnivore Diet.

5. **Hydration and Electrolytes:** During fasting periods, it's important to stay hydrated and maintain electrolyte balance. Drinking water and consuming electrolyte-rich beverages such as bone broth or salted water can help prevent dehydration and support overall well-being. Adequate hydration and electrolyte intake are especially important when practicing extended fasting.

Fasting and intermittent feeding strategies can complement the Carnivore Diet by promoting fat adaptation, improving metabolic flexibility, and enhancing overall health. Individuals interested in incorporating fasting into their Carnivore Diet should start gradually, listen to their body's hunger cues, and consult with a healthcare professional if needed, especially if they have underlying health conditions or concerns. With careful planning and attention to hydration and electrolytes, fasting can be safely integrated into the Carnivore Diet to support optimal health and well-being.

Adaptation Period: What to Expect When Transitioning

Transitioning to the Carnivore Diet can be a significant dietary shift for many individuals, and it often involves an adaptation period as the body adjusts to the new eating pattern. Here's what to expect during the adaptation period:

1. **Initial Changes in Digestive Function:** As the body adapts to the Carnivore Diet, some individuals may experience changes in digestive function, including alterations in bowel habits, such as constipation or diarrhea. This is commonly referred to as the "Carnivore Flu" or "Keto Flu" and may be accompanied by symptoms such as fatigue, headache, and irritability. These symptoms are typically temporary and tend to subside as the body adjusts to the new dietary regimen.

2. **Transitioning to Fat Metabolism:** The Carnivore Diet promotes fat adaptation, where the body becomes more efficient at using fat for fuel in the absence of carbohydrates. During the adaptation period, individuals may experience fluctuations in energy levels and appetite as the body transitions from relying on carbohydrates to utilizing fat for energy. Some people may notice an initial decrease in energy or performance during physical activities, but this often improves over time as fat adaptation occurs.

3. **Changes in Food Cravings and Preferences:** As individuals transition to the Carnivore Diet, they may experience changes in food cravings and preferences. Cravings for sugary or processed foods may diminish as the body becomes accustomed to a diet based primarily on animal foods. Some individuals may also notice changes in taste perception, with a heightened appreciation for the flavors and textures of meat, fish, and other animal-based foods.

4. **Adjustment Period for Digestive System:** The Carnivore Diet eliminates many common dietary irritants found in plant-based foods, which can lead to improvements in digestive health for some individuals. However, it may take time for the digestive system to adjust to the higher intake of animal-based foods, particularly if transitioning from a diet high in fiber. Incorporating bone broth, fermented foods, and other gut-supportive foods can help promote digestive health and ease the transition.

5. **Monitoring Nutrient Intake:** During the adaptation period, it's important to monitor nutrient intake and ensure adequate hydration and electrolyte balance. Some individuals may benefit from supplementation with vitamins and minerals, particularly during the initial stages of the Carnivore Diet. Consulting with a healthcare professional or registered dietitian can help identify any potential nutrient deficiencies and provide personalized recommendations for optimizing nutrient intake on the Carnivore Diet.

Overall, the adaptation period when transitioning to the Carnivore Diet can vary from person to person, with some individuals experiencing minimal discomfort while others may encounter more pronounced symptoms. Patience, perseverance, and attention to individual needs and preferences are key during this period of adjustment. With time, many individuals find that they adapt well to the Carnivore Diet and experience improvements in energy levels, mental clarity, and overall well-being.

Chapter 3
Getting Started: Preparing for Success

Welcome to the carnivore diet, a dietary approach that focuses on consuming animal products exclusively. Whether you're considering this lifestyle for health reasons, weight loss, or performance enhancement, proper preparation is key to success. In this cookbook, we'll outline essential steps to help you embark on your carnivore journey confidently.

The carnivore diet is based on the principle of eating animal-derived foods while excluding plant-based foods. This includes meat, fish, eggs, and certain dairy products like butter and cheese. The primary goal is to eliminate all plant foods, including grains, fruits, vegetables, legumes, and processed foods.

Before Starting:

1. Consult a Healthcare Professional: Before making any significant dietary changes, it's crucial to consult with a healthcare professional, especially if you have underlying health conditions or concerns.

2. Educate Yourself: Research the carnivore diet extensively to understand its principles, potential benefits, and possible risks. Consider reading books, scientific articles, and reputable online sources.

3. Set Clear Goals: Determine your reasons for adopting the carnivore diet. Whether it's weight loss, improved energy levels, or better health markers, setting clear goals will keep you motivated and focused.

Transitioning to the Carnivore Diet:

1. Gradual Transition: For some individuals, transitioning abruptly to a carnivore diet can lead to digestive discomfort. Consider gradually reducing your intake of plant foods while increasing animal-based foods over a period of days or weeks.

2. Stock Up on Essentials: Prioritize high-quality animal products such as grass-fed beef, pasture-raised poultry, wild-caught fish, and organic eggs. Having a well-stocked kitchen will make it easier to stick to your carnivore diet.

3. Experiment with Food Varieties: Explore different cuts of meat, cooking methods, and seasoning options to keep your meals exciting and satisfying. Embrace variety within the confines of animal-based foods.

Meal Planning and Preparation:

1. Plan Your Meals: Take time to plan your carnivore meals to ensure you're getting a balanced intake of nutrients. Include a variety of animal proteins, fats, and organs to meet your body's needs.

2. Batch Cooking: Consider batch cooking large quantities of meat and storing them for easy access throughout the week. This will save you time and effort while ensuring you always have carnivore-friendly options on hand.

3. Embrace Simplicity: Carnivore meals can be simple yet delicious. Focus on high-quality ingredients prepared with minimal seasoning and processing. Experiment with different cooking techniques, such as grilling, roasting, and slow cooking, to enhance flavour and texture.

Navigating Challenges:

1. Addressing Cravings: As you transition to the carnivore diet, you may experience cravings for familiar plant-based foods. Stay committed to your

goals and remind yourself of the reasons why you chose this dietary approach.

2. Managing Social Situations: Eating a carnivore diet may present challenges in social settings where plant-based options are prevalent. Communicate your dietary preferences politely and be prepared to make adjustments when dining out or attending social gatherings.

3. Monitoring Health Markers: Keep track of your health markers, including energy levels, digestion, weight, and any changes in existing health conditions. If you notice any adverse effects, consult with a healthcare professional to make necessary adjustments.

Assessing Your Goals and Motivations

Before embarking on any significant journey, it's essential to take a step back and assess your goals and motivations. This holds true, especially when considering dietary changes like adopting the carnivore diet. Understanding why you want to pursue this lifestyle and what you hope to achieve will provide clarity and direction throughout your journey. Let's delve into the process of assessing your goals and motivations for adopting the carnivore diet.

1. **Reflect on Your Health Objectives:**

    - Begin by reflecting on your current health status and any specific health goals you aim to achieve. Are you looking to improve your energy levels, manage weight, enhance athletic performance, or address certain health conditions?

    - Consider how the carnivore diet aligns with your health objectives. Research the potential benefits of this dietary approach and evaluate whether it addresses your specific health concerns or goals.

2. **Examine Your Relationship with Food:**

    - Take a closer look at your relationship with food and your eating habits. Are there certain foods or dietary patterns that you feel negatively impact your health or well-being?

    - Assess whether the carnivore diet offers a solution to any challenges or issues you experience with food. Determine if the simplicity and restriction of the carnivore diet resonate with your preferences and lifestyle.

3. **Identify Your Motivations:**

- Explore the underlying motivations driving your interest in the carnivore diet. Are you intrigued by the potential health benefits, inspired by success stories, or seeking a new dietary challenge?

- Dig deeper to uncover personal reasons behind your desire to adopt the carnivore diet. Whether it's curiosity, a desire for self-improvement, or a quest for optimal health, understanding your motivations will fuel your commitment and determination.

4. **Set Clear and Realistic Goals**:

- Based on your reflections and motivations, set clear and realistic goals for your carnivore journey. Define specific, measurable, and achievable outcomes that you hope to attain.

- Consider both short-term and long-term goals, allowing yourself to celebrate milestones along the way while staying focused on the bigger picture.

5. **Evaluate Your Readiness:**

- Assess your readiness to embrace the carnivore diet based on your goals, motivations, and current circumstances. Are you mentally prepared to commit to this dietary approach and navigate potential challenges?

- Consider any practical considerations, such as access to high-quality animal products, support from healthcare professionals, and social support from friends and family.

Kitchen Essentials for Carnivore Cooking

Embarking on the carnivore diet requires a well-equipped kitchen to support your culinary endeavours. Whether you're a seasoned carnivore or new to this dietary approach, having the right tools and equipment can make meal preparation more efficient and enjoyable. In this cookbook, we'll explore essential kitchen essentials for carnivore cooking, helping you create delicious and satisfying meals cantered around animal-based foods.

1. **High-Quality Meat:**

    - Prioritize high-quality cuts of meat, such as grass-fed beef, pasture-raised poultry, wild-caught fish, and organ meats. Choose fresh, organic options whenever possible to ensure optimal taste and nutritional value.

2. **Sharp Knives:**

    - Invest in a set of sharp knives suitable for various cutting tasks, including slicing, chopping, and deboning meat. Sharp knives make food preparation safer and more precise, allowing you to easily handle different cuts of meat.

3. **Meat Thermometer:**

    - A meat thermometer is essential for ensuring your meat is cooked to the desired level of doneness and safe for consumption. Invest in a reliable digital thermometer with instant-read capabilities for accurate temperature readings.

4. **Cast Iron Skillet or Grill:**

- A cast iron skillet or grill is versatile and ideal for cooking meat on the carnivore diet. Whether you're searing steaks, grilling chicken, or frying bacon, cast iron provides excellent heat retention and creates a beautiful sear on your meats.

5. **Roasting Pan:**

- A roasting pan is essential for cooking larger cuts of meat, such as whole chickens, roasts, or ribs. Look for a durable roasting pan with a rack to elevate the meat and allow air to circulate evenly for thorough cooking.

6. **Slow Cooker or Instant Pot:**

- Slow cookers and Instant Pots are convenient appliances for preparing tender and flavorful meat dishes with minimal effort. Use them to cook stews, soups, and braised meats, allowing you to enjoy delicious carnivore meals with minimal hands-on time.

7. **Food Processor or Meat Grinder:**

- A food processor or meat grinder is useful for grinding meat, making homemade sausages, and preparing meat-based sauces or spreads. Choose a sturdy and reliable appliance capable of handling different textures and quantities of meat.

8. **Cutting Board:**

- Invest in a durable and easy-to-clean cutting board dedicated to meat preparation. Opt for a non-porous material, such as plastic or bamboo, to prevent cross-contamination and maintain food safety.

9. **Quality Seasonings and Spices:**

- While the carnivore diet primarily focuses on animal-based foods, adding quality seasonings and spices can enhance the flavor of your meals. Stock up on staples like salt, pepper, garlic powder, and dried herbs to season your meat dishes to perfection.

10. Storage Containers:

- Keep your carnivore meals fresh and organized with a selection of storage containers. Choose containers that are freezer-safe, microwave-safe, and stackable for easy storage and reheating of leftovers.

Grocery Shopping and Meal Planning Tips

Effective grocery shopping and meal planning are essential components of success on the carnivore diet. By carefully selecting high-quality animal products and planning your meals in advance, you can ensure that you have the necessary ingredients on hand to support your dietary goals. In this cookbook, we'll provide practical tips to streamline your grocery shopping and meal planning process, making it easier to adhere to the carnivore lifestyle.

1. **Plan Your Meals:**

   - Before heading to the grocery store, take time to plan your meals for the week. Consider your schedule, dietary preferences, and nutritional needs when selecting recipes and organizing your meal plan.

   - Aim for a balance of protein, fats, and organs in each meal to ensure you're meeting your body's nutritional requirements on the carnivore diet.

2. **Make a Shopping List:**

   - Based on your meal plan, create a comprehensive shopping list of the animal products and essentials you'll need for the week. Organize your list by category (e.g., meat, poultry, eggs, dairy) to make shopping more efficient.

   - Include any seasonings, spices, or condiments you'll need to flavor your meals, as well as household staples like cooking oil and salt.

3. **Choose High-Quality Animal Products:**

- When selecting meat, poultry, fish, and dairy products, prioritize high-quality, minimally processed options. Look for grass-fed beef, pasture-raised poultry, wild-caught fish, and organic eggs to maximize nutritional value and flavor.

- Consider purchasing in bulk or visiting local farmers' markets for fresh, locally sourced animal products.

4. Explore Variety:

- Embrace variety within the carnivore diet by incorporating different cuts of meat, types of seafood, and organ meats into your meals. Experiment with cooking methods and seasonings to keep your meals interesting and satisfying.

- Don't hesitate to try new recipes and explore traditional dishes from various cultures that feature animal-based ingredients.

5. Stock Up on Staples:

- In addition to fresh animal products, stock up on staple items that will support your carnivore lifestyle. These may include cooking fats (e.g., butter, tallow, lard), bone broth, gelatin, and collagen supplements.

- Consider purchasing non-perishable items in bulk to save money and ensure you always have essentials on hand.

6. Shop Mindfully:

- When grocery shopping, stick to your list and avoid impulse purchases of non-carnivore foods. Pay attention to food labels and ingredients to ensure that the products you're purchasing align with your dietary goals.

- Take advantage of sales and discounts on animal products to maximize savings without compromising quality.

7. **Meal Prep for Success:**

- Set aside time each week for meal prep to streamline your carnivore cooking and save time during busy weekdays. Cook large batches of meat, poultry, and eggs, and portion them into individual servings for easy grab-and-go meals.

- Consider preparing marinades, sauces, and seasoning blends in advance to add flavor and variety to your carnivore dishes throughout the week.

Tracking Progress and Adjusting as Needed

Tracking your progress and making adjustments along the way are essential components of success on the carnivore diet. Whether you're pursuing health improvements, weight loss, or performance goals, monitoring key indicators allows you to assess your journey's effectiveness and make informed decisions about your dietary approach. In this cookbook, we'll explore strategies for tracking progress and adjusting as needed on the carnivore diet.

1. **Establish Baseline Measurements:**

    - Before starting the carnivore diet, establish baseline measurements of relevant health markers, such as weight, body composition, blood pressure, and blood glucose levels. These initial measurements will serve as reference points for tracking progress over time.

2. **Track Dietary Intake:**

    - Keep a record of your daily dietary intake, including types and quantities of animal products consumed. This may involve using a food journal, mobile app, or online tracking tool to log meals and monitor nutrient intake.

    - Pay attention to macronutrient ratios, such as protein, fat, and carbohydrate content, to ensure you're meeting your nutritional needs on the carnivore diet.

3. **Monitor Health Indicators:**

    - Regularly assess key health indicators to gauge the impact of the carnivore diet on your overall health and well-being. These may include energy levels, digestion, sleep quality, mood, and cognitive function.

- Track any changes in existing health conditions or symptoms, such as inflammation, joint pain, allergies, or autoimmune issues, to determine how the carnivore diet is influencing your health.

4. **Assess Performance and Fitness:**

   - If you're incorporating the carnivore diet as part of a fitness or athletic regimen, track performance metrics relevant to your goals. This may include strength, endurance, speed, agility, and recovery time.

   - Evaluate changes in body composition, muscle mass, and physical performance to determine the effectiveness of the carnivore diet in supporting your fitness objectives.

5. **Listen to Your Body:**

   - Pay close attention to your body's signals and feedback as you follow the carnivore diet. Notice how you feel before, during, and after meals, as well as any changes in hunger, satiety, cravings, and energy levels.

   - Trust your instincts and intuition when it comes to adjusting your dietary approach based on your body's responses and needs.

6. **Make Informed Adjustments:**

   - Based on your progress tracking and observations, make informed adjustments to your dietary approach as needed. This may involve fine-tuning your macronutrient ratios, experimenting with different types of animal products, or incorporating supplements to address nutritional deficiencies.

- Consult with healthcare professionals or nutrition experts for personalized guidance and recommendations tailored to your individual goals and health status.

7. Stay Flexible and Adaptive:

- Recognize that dietary needs and responses can vary among individuals, and what works for one person may not necessarily work for another. Stay open-minded and willing to adjust your approach based on feedback from your body and ongoing progress tracking.

Embrace a mindset of continuous learning and adaptation as you navigate your carnivore journey, striving for optimal health and well-being over the long term.

Chapter 4
Basics Recipes

Ribeye Steak

Cooking Time: 10 minutes

Servings: 1

Nutritional Information: 600 calories, 50g protein, 0g carbohydrates, 0g fiber, 45g fat

Ingredients:

- 1 Ribeye steak (8 oz)

- Salt and pepper to taste

Instructions:

1. Preheat a grill or skillet over medium-high heat.

2. Season the ribeye steak generously with salt and pepper on both sides.

3. Place the steak on the grill or skillet and cook for about 4-5 minutes on each side for medium-rare, or until desired doneness is reached.

4. Let the steak rest for a few minutes before slicing.

5. Serve hot.

Helpful Tip: Allow the steak to come to room temperature before cooking for more even cooking.

Baked Salmon

Cooking Time: 15 minutes

Servings: 1

Nutritional Information: 350 calories, 40g protein, 0g carbohydrates, 0g fiber, 20g fat

Ingredients:

- 1 Salmon fillet (6 oz)

- Salt and pepper to taste

Instructions:

1. Preheat the oven to 400°F (200°C).

2. Place the salmon fillet on a baking sheet lined with parchment paper.

3. Season the salmon with salt and pepper.

4. Bake for 12-15 minutes, or until the salmon is cooked through and flakes easily with a fork.

5. Serve hot.

Helpful Tip: Brush the salmon with butter or olive oil for added flavor and moisture.

Beef Burger Patties

Cooking Time: 8 minutes

Servings: 1

Nutritional Information: 400 calories, 30g protein, 0g carbohydrates, 0g fiber, 30g fat

Ingredients:

- 1/2 lb ground beef

- Salt and pepper to taste

Instructions:

1. Preheat a grill or skillet over medium-high heat.

2. Divide the ground beef into two equal portions and shape into burger patties.

3. Season both sides of the patties with salt and pepper.

4. Cook the patties for about 3-4 minutes on each side, or until they reach the desired level of doneness.

5. Serve hot, optionally with your choice of condiments.

Helpful Tip: Use high-fat ground beef for juicier burgers.

Grilled Chicken Thighs

Cooking Time: 15 minutes

Servings: 1

Nutritional Information: 400 calories, 30g protein, 0g carbohydrates, 0g fiber, 30g fat

Ingredients:

- 2 Chicken thighs (bone-in, skin-on)

- Salt and pepper to taste

Instructions:

1. Preheat a grill to medium heat.

2. Season the chicken thighs with salt and pepper on both sides.

3. Place the chicken thighs on the grill, skin side down, and cook for about 6-8 minutes.

4. Flip the chicken thighs and continue cooking for another 6-8 minutes, or until the internal temperature reaches 165°F (75°C).

5. Serve hot.

Helpful Tip: Marinate the chicken thighs for extra flavor before grilling.

Pan-Seared Duck Breast

Cooking Time: 15 minutes

Servings: 1

Nutritional Information: 450 calories, 25g protein, 0g carbohydrates, 0g fiber, 40g fat

Ingredients:

- 1 Duck breast (6 oz)
- Salt and pepper to taste

Instructions:

1. Score the skin of the duck breast with a sharp knife in a criss-cross pattern.

2. Season both sides of the duck breast generously with salt and pepper.

3. Place the duck breast skin-side down in a cold skillet.

4. Turn the heat to medium-high and cook for about 8-10 minutes, rendering the fat from the skin until it becomes crispy.

5. Flip the duck breast and cook for an additional 3-5 minutes on the other side, or until desired doneness is reached.

6. Let the duck breast rest for a few minutes before slicing.

7. Serve hot.

Helpful Tip: Save the rendered duck fat for cooking vegetables or for added flavor in other dishes.

Grilled Pork Chops

Cooking Time: 12 minutes

Servings: 1

Nutritional Information: 400 calories, 35g protein, 0g carbohydrates, 0g fiber, 30g fat

Ingredients:

- 1 Pork chop (bone-in, 8 oz)

- Salt and pepper to taste

Instructions:

1. Preheat a grill to medium-high heat.

2. Season the pork chop with salt and pepper on both sides.

3. Place the pork chop on the grill and cook for about 5-6 minutes on each side, or until the internal temperature reaches 145°F (63°C).

4. Remove from the grill and let it rest for a few minutes before serving.

5. Serve hot.

Helpful Tip: Brine the pork chop beforehand for extra juiciness and flavor.

Lamb Chops with Rosemary

Cooking Time: 10 minutes

Servings: 1

Nutritional Information: 500 calories, 25g protein, 0g carbohydrates, 0g fiber, 40g fat

Ingredients:

- 2 Lamb chops (4 oz each)

- Salt and pepper to taste

- Fresh rosemary sprigs

Instructions:

1. Preheat a grill or skillet over medium-high heat.

2. Season the lamb chops with salt and pepper on both sides.

3. Place a fresh rosemary sprig on top of each lamb chop.

4. Grill or sear the lamb chops for about 4-5 minutes on each side for medium-rare, or adjust cooking time according to desired doneness.

5. Remove from heat and let the lamb chops rest for a few minutes before serving.

6. Discard the rosemary sprigs before serving.

7. Serve hot.

Helpful Tip: Lamb pairs well with mint sauce or a squeeze of lemon juice for added flavor.

Seared Tuna Steaks

Cooking Time: 6 minutes

Servings: 1

Nutritional Information: 300 calories, 40g protein, 0g carbohydrates, 0g fiber, 15g fat

Ingredients:

- 1 Tuna steak (6 oz)

- Salt and pepper to taste

- Sesame seeds (optional)

Instructions:

1. Heat a skillet over high heat.

2. Season the tuna steak with salt and pepper on both sides.

3. If desired, coat the edges of the tuna steak with sesame seeds.

4. Sear the tuna steak for about 1-2 minutes on each side for rare to medium-rare doneness, depending on thickness.

5. Remove from the skillet and let it rest for a minute.

6. Slice thinly against the grain before serving.

7. Serve hot.

Helpful Tip: Serve the seared tuna steak with soy sauce or wasabi for dipping.

Pan-Fried Venison Steak

Cooking Time: 10 minutes

Servings: 1

Nutritional Information: 350 calories, 50g protein, 0g carbohydrates, 0g fiber, 15g fat

Ingredients:

- 1 Venison steak (6 oz)

- Salt and pepper to taste

- Butter or cooking fat of choice

Instructions:

1. Heat a skillet over medium-high heat and add butter or cooking fat.

2. Season the venison steak with salt and pepper on both sides.

3. Place the steak in the skillet and cook for about 3-4 minutes on each side for medium-rare, or adjust cooking time according to desired doneness.

4. Remove the steak from the skillet and let it rest for a few minutes before slicing.

5. Serve hot.

Helpful Tip: Avoid overcooking venison as it can become tough. Aim for medium-rare for the best flavor and tenderness.

10. Pan-Seared Duck Legs

Cooking Time: 20 minutes

Servings: 1

Nutritional Information: 550 calories, 30g protein, 0g carbohydrates, 0g fiber, 45g fat

Ingredients:

- 2 Duck legs

- Salt and pepper to taste

- Duck fat or cooking fat of choice

Instructions:

1. Preheat the oven to 350°F (175°C).

2. Heat a skillet over medium-high heat and add duck fat or cooking fat.

3. Season the duck legs with salt and pepper.

4. Sear the duck legs in the skillet, skin side down, until golden brown, about 4-5 minutes.

5. Flip the duck legs and sear the other side for another 4-5 minutes.

6. Transfer the duck legs to a baking dish and roast in the preheated oven for 10-12 minutes, or until fully cooked.

7. Serve hot.

Helpful Tip: Save the rendered duck fat for cooking or roasting vegetables for added flavor.

Pan-Seared Beef Liver

Cooking Time: 8 minutes

Servings: 1

Nutritional Information: 250 calories, 30g protein, 0g carbohydrates, 0g fiber, 15g fat

Ingredients:

- 4 oz Beef liver, sliced

- Salt and pepper to taste

- 2 tbsp Butter or cooking fat of choice

Instructions:

1. Heat a skillet over medium-high heat and add butter or cooking fat.

2. Season the beef liver slices with salt and pepper on both sides.

3. Place the liver slices in the skillet and sear for about 2-3 minutes on each side, or until cooked through but still pink in the center.

4. Avoid overcooking to prevent toughness.

5. Remove from the skillet and let rest for a minute before serving.

6. Serve hot.

Helpful Tip: Soak the beef liver in milk for 30 minutes before cooking to help reduce bitterness.

Bacon-Wrapped Chicken Tenders

Cooking Time: 20 minutes

Servings: 1

Nutritional Information: 400 calories, 35g protein, 0g carbohydrates, 0g fiber, 30g fat

Ingredients:

- 4 Chicken tenders

- 4 slices Bacon

- Salt and pepper to taste

Instructions:

1. Preheat the oven to 400°F (200°C).

2. Season the chicken tenders with salt and pepper.

3. Wrap each chicken tender with a slice of bacon.

4. Place the bacon-wrapped chicken tenders on a baking sheet lined with parchment paper.

5. Bake in the preheated oven for 15-20 minutes, or until the bacon is crispy and the chicken is cooked through.

6. Serve hot.

Helpful Tip: Secure the bacon with toothpicks to prevent unwrapping during cooking.

Chapter 5
Red Meat Recipes

Beef Rib Roast

Cooking Time: 2 hours 30 minutes

Servings: 4

Ingredients:

- 1 (4-pound) beef rib roast

- Salt and pepper to taste

Instructions:

1. Preheat the oven to 350°F (175°C).

2. Season the beef rib roast generously with salt and pepper.

3. Place the roast in a roasting pan, fat side up.

4. Roast in the preheated oven for about 2 to 2 ½ hours, or until the internal temperature reaches 135°F (57°C) for medium-rare.

5. Remove from the oven and let it rest for 10-15 minutes before slicing.

6. Serve hot.

Nutritional Information: 400 calories, 50g protein, 0g carbohydrates, 0g fiber, 20g fat

Helpful Tip: Use a meat thermometer to ensure accurate cooking temperatures for the desired level of doneness.

Beef Stew

Cooking Time: 2 hours

Servings: 4

Ingredients:

- 2 pounds beef chuck, cut into cubes

- Salt and pepper to taste

- 2 tablespoons cooking fat (e.g., tallow, lard)

- 4 cups beef broth

Instructions:

1. Season the beef cubes with salt and pepper.

2. Heat the cooking fat in a large pot over medium-high heat.

3. Brown the beef cubes on all sides in batches, then set aside.

4. Once all the beef is browned, return it to the pot and add beef broth.

5. Bring to a boil, then reduce heat to low and simmer, covered, for about 1 ½ to 2 hours, or until the beef is tender.

6. Serve hot.

Nutritional Information: 350 calories, 40g protein, 0g carbohydrates, 0g fiber, 20g fat

Helpful Tip: Add herbs and spices for extra flavor, such as rosemary, thyme, or garlic.

Grilled Lamb Chops

Cooking Time: 10 minutes

Servings: 2

Ingredients:

- 4 Lamb chops

- Salt and pepper to taste

Instructions:

1. Preheat the grill to medium-high heat.

2. Season the lamb chops with salt and pepper on both sides.

3. Place the lamb chops on the grill and cook for about 3-4 minutes on each side for medium-rare, or adjust cooking time according to desired doneness.

4. Remove from the grill and let them rest for a few minutes before serving.

5. Serve hot.

Nutritional Information: 450 calories, 50g protein, 0g carbohydrates, 0g fiber, 25g fat

Helpful Tip: For added flavor, marinate the lamb chops in olive oil, garlic, and herbs before grilling.

Beef Liver Pâté

Cooking Time: 30 minutes

Servings: 8

Ingredients:

- 1 lb beef liver, trimmed
- 1 onion, chopped
- 2 cloves garlic, minced
- 1/2 cup beef broth
- 1/4 cup butter

Instructions:

1. In a skillet, melt butter over medium heat. Add onions and garlic and sauté until soft.

2. Add beef liver to the skillet and cook until browned on both sides, about 3-4 minutes per side.

3. Transfer the liver, onions, and garlic to a food processor. Add beef broth and process until smooth.

4. Season with salt and pepper to taste.

5. Transfer the pâté to a serving dish or ramekins and refrigerate until firm.

6. Serve chilled.

Nutritional Information: 200 calories, 20g protein, 2g carbohydrates, 0g fiber, 12g fat

Helpful Tip: Serve with sliced cucumber or celery sticks for a crunchy texture.

Beef Brisket

Cooking Time: 4 hours

Servings: 6

Ingredients:

- 3-4 pounds beef brisket

- Salt and pepper to taste

- 2 cups beef broth

Instructions:

1. Preheat the oven to 300°F (150°C).

2. Season the beef brisket generously with salt and pepper on both sides.

3. Place the brisket in a roasting pan and pour beef broth over it.

4. Cover the roasting pan with foil and roast in the preheated oven for about 3 ½ to 4 hours, or until the brisket is tender.

5. Remove from the oven and let it rest for 10-15 minutes before slicing.

6. Serve hot.

Nutritional Information: 300 calories, 40g protein, 0g carbohydrates, 0g fibre, 15g fat

Helpful Tip: For extra flavour, rub the brisket with a dry spice rub before roasting.

Beef Short Ribs

Cooking Time: 3 hours

Servings: 4

Ingredients:

- 2 pounds beef short ribs

- Salt and pepper to taste

- 2 cups beef broth

Instructions:

1. Preheat the oven to 325°F (160°C).

2. Season the beef short ribs with salt and pepper on all sides.

3. Place the short ribs in a roasting pan and pour beef broth over them.

4. Cover the roasting pan with foil and roast in the preheated oven for about 2 ½ to 3 hours, or until the short ribs are tender and falling off the bone.

5. Remove from the oven and let them rest for a few minutes before serving.

6. Serve hot.

Nutritional Information: 400 calories, 40g protein, 0g carbohydrates, 0g fiber, 25g fat

Helpful Tip: For a caramelized crust, sear the short ribs in a hot skillet before roasting.

Beef Kabobs

Cooking Time: 20 minutes

Servings: 4

Ingredients:

- 1 lb beef sirloin, cut into cubes

- Salt and pepper to taste

- Wooden or metal skewers

Instructions:

1. Preheat the grill to medium-high heat.

2. Season the beef cubes with salt and pepper.

3. Thread the beef cubes onto skewers.

4. Grill the kabobs for about 8-10 minutes, turning occasionally, until the beef is cooked to desired doneness.

5. Remove from the grill and let them rest for a few minutes before serving.

6. Serve hot.

Nutritional Information: 350 calories, 40g protein, 0g carbohydrates, 0g fiber, 20g fat

Helpful Tip: Add chunks of bell peppers or onions to the skewers for added flavour and variety.

Beef Bourguignon

Cooking Time: 2 hours 30 minutes

Servings: 6

Ingredients:

- 2 lbs beef chuck, cut into cubes

- Salt and pepper to taste

- 4 slices bacon, chopped

- 1 onion, chopped

- 2 cloves garlic, minced

- 2 cups beef broth

- 1 cup red wine

- 2 tbsp tomato paste

- Fresh thyme and parsley, for garnish

Instructions:

1. Season the beef cubes with salt and pepper.

2. In a large pot or Dutch oven, cook the chopped bacon over medium heat until crispy.

3. Remove the bacon from the pot and set aside, leaving the bacon fat in the pot.

4. Brown the beef cubes in the bacon fat in batches, then set aside.

5. Add the chopped onion and minced garlic to the pot and sauté until softened.

6. Return the beef cubes and bacon to the pot. Add beef broth, red wine, and tomato paste. Bring to a simmer.

7. Cover and simmer over low heat for about 2 hours, or until the beef is tender.

8. Serve hot, garnished with fresh thyme and parsley.

Nutritional Information: 400 calories, 35g protein, 5g carbohydrates, 1g fiber, 25g fat

Helpful Tip: Serve over cauliflower rice or enjoy on its own for a hearty meal.

Beef Ribs

Cooking Time: 3 hours 30 minutes

Servings: 4

Ingredients:

- 2 racks beef ribs

- Barbecue sauce (optional)

Instructions:

1. Preheat the oven to 300°F (150°C).

2. Season the beef ribs with salt and pepper on both sides.

3. Place the ribs on a baking sheet lined with aluminum foil.

4. Cover the ribs tightly with another sheet of foil.

5. Bake in the preheated oven for about 3 to 3 ½ hours, or until the meat is tender and easily pulls away from the bone.

6. Optionally, brush the ribs with barbecue sauce during the last 30 minutes of cooking.

7. Remove from the oven and let them rest for a few minutes before serving.

8. Serve hot.

Nutritional Information: 450 calories, 40g protein, 0g carbohydrates, 0g fiber, 30g fat

Helpful Tip: For a smoky flavor, you can also cook the ribs on a grill or smoker.

Beef Liver Steak

Cooking Time: 10 minutes

Servings: 2

Ingredients:

- 1 lb beef liver, sliced

- Salt and pepper to taste

- Butter or cooking fat of choice

Instructions:

1. Heat a skillet over medium-high heat and add butter or cooking fat.

2. Season the beef liver slices with salt and pepper on both sides.

3. Place the liver slices in the skillet and cook for about 2-3 minutes on each side, or until cooked through but still pink in the center.

4. Avoid overcooking to prevent toughness.

5. Remove from the skillet and let rest for a minute before serving.

6. Serve hot.

Nutritional Information: 350 calories, 30g protein, 0g carbohydrates, 0g fiber, 25g fat

Helpful Tip: Soaking the beef liver in milk before cooking can help reduce bitterness.

Beef Tenderloin Steak

Cooking Time: 10 minutes

Servings: 2

Ingredients:

- 2 Beef tenderloin steaks (6 oz each)

- Salt and pepper to taste

- Butter or cooking fat of choice

Instructions:

1. Preheat a skillet over medium-high heat and add butter or cooking fat.

2. Season the beef tenderloin steaks with salt and pepper on both sides.

3. Place the steaks in the skillet and cook for about 3-4 minutes on each side for medium-rare, or adjust cooking time according to desired doneness.

4. Remove from the skillet and let them rest for a few minutes before serving.

5. Serve hot.

Nutritional Information: 450 calories, 50g protein, 0g carbohydrates, 0g fiber, 25g fat

Helpful Tip: For added flavor, rub the steaks with minced garlic or your favorite steak seasoning before cooking.

Beef Shawarma

Cooking Time: 20 minutes

Servings: 4

Ingredients:

- 1 lb beef sirloin, thinly sliced
- 2 tablespoons olive oil
- 2 cloves garlic, minced
- 1 teaspoon ground cumin
- 1 teaspoon paprika
- 1/2 teaspoon ground turmeric
- 1/2 teaspoon ground cinnamon

Instructions:

1. In a bowl, combine the sliced beef, olive oil, minced garlic, cumin, paprika, turmeric, cinnamon, salt, and pepper. Mix well to coat the beef evenly.

2. Heat a skillet over medium-high heat and add the marinated beef slices.

3. Cook for about 5-7 minutes, stirring occasionally, until the beef is cooked through and slightly crispy on the edges.

4. Serve hot.

Nutritional Information: 300 calories, 35g protein, 1g carbohydrates, 0g fiber, 15g fat

Helpful Tip: Serve the beef shawarma with a side of tzatziki sauce and lettuce wraps for a low-carb meal option.

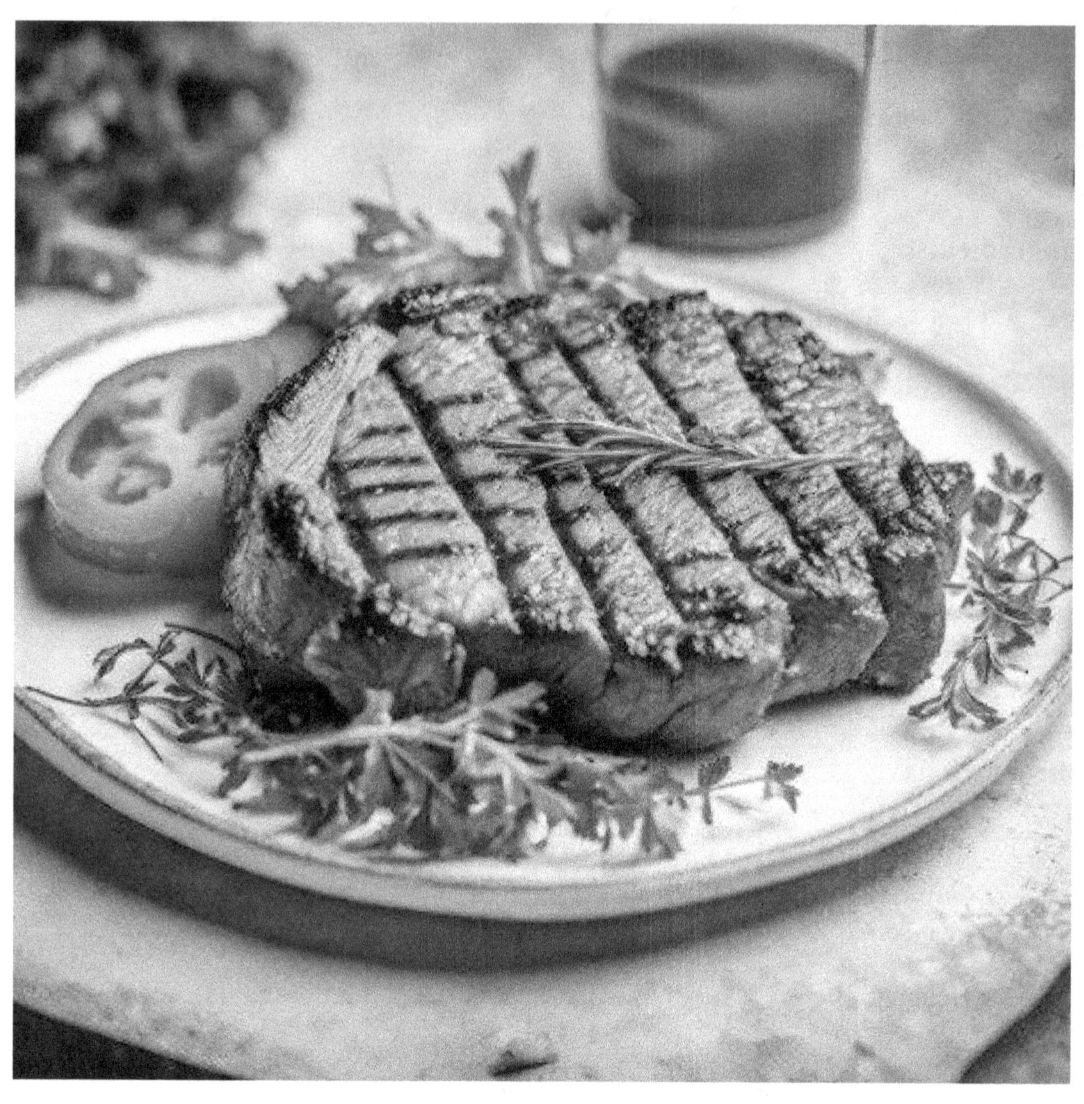

Chapter 6
Pork and Poultry

Roast Chicken

Cooking Time: 1 hour 30 minutes

Servings: 4

Ingredients:

- 1 whole chicken (about 4 pounds)

Instructions:

1. Preheat the oven to 375°F (190°C).

2. Rinse the chicken under cold water and pat dry with paper towels.

3. Season the chicken generously with salt and pepper, both inside and out.

4. Place the chicken breast-side up in a roasting pan.

5. Roast in the preheated oven for about 1 hour and 15 minutes to 1 hour and 30 minutes, or until the internal temperature reaches 165°F (75°C).

6. Remove from the oven and let it rest for 10-15 minutes before carving.

7. Serve hot.

Nutritional Information: 250 calories, 30g protein, 0g carbohydrates, 0g fiber, 15g fat

Helpful Tip: For crispy skin, pat the chicken dry with paper towels before seasoning and roasting.

Grilled Pork Tenderloin

Cooking Time: 20 minutes

Servings: 4

Ingredients:

- 2 pork tenderloins (about 1 pound each)

- Salt and pepper to taste

Instructions:

1. Preheat the grill to medium-high heat.

2. Season the pork tenderloins with salt and pepper on all sides.

3. Place the tenderloins on the grill and cook for about 8-10 minutes per side, or until the internal temperature reaches 145°F (63°C).

4. Remove from the grill and let them rest for a few minutes before slicing.

5. Serve hot.

Nutritional Information: 200 calories, 25g protein, 0g carbohydrates, 0g fiber, 10g fat

Helpful Tip: For added flavor, marinate the pork tenderloins in your favorite marinade for a few hours before grilling.

Bacon-Wrapped Chicken Thighs

Cooking Time: 30 minutes

Servings: 4

Ingredients:

- 8 boneless, skinless chicken thighs

- 8 slices bacon

- Salt and pepper to taste

Instructions:

1. Preheat the oven to 400°F (200°C).

2. Season the chicken thighs with salt and pepper.

3. Wrap each chicken thigh with a slice of bacon, securing it with toothpicks if necessary.

4. Place the bacon-wrapped chicken thighs on a baking sheet lined with parchment paper.

5. Bake in the preheated oven for 25-30 minutes, or until the chicken is cooked through and the bacon is crispy.

6. Remove from the oven and let them rest for a few minutes before serving.

7. Serve hot.

Nutritional Information: 300 calories, 30g protein, 0g carbohydrates, 0g fiber, 20g fat

Helpful Tip: Broil for a few minutes at the end of cooking for extra crispiness.

Pork Chops with Garlic Butter

Cooking Time: 20 minutes

Servings: 4

Ingredients:

- 4 pork chops (about 1 inch thick)

- 4 tablespoons unsalted butter

- 4 cloves garlic, minced

Instructions:

1. Season the pork chops with salt and pepper on both sides.

2. Heat a skillet over medium-high heat and add 2 tablespoons of butter.

3. Add the minced garlic to the skillet and cook until fragrant, about 1 minute.

4. Place the pork chops in the skillet and cook for about 4-5 minutes on each side, or until golden brown and cooked through.

5. Add the remaining 2 tablespoons of butter to the skillet during the last minute of cooking.

6. Baste the pork chops with the melted garlic butter.

7. Remove from the skillet and let them rest for a few minutes before serving.

8. Serve hot.

Nutritional Information: 350 calories, 30g protein, 0g carbohydrates, 0g fiber, 25g fat

Helpful Tip: Use bone-in pork chops for extra flavor and juiciness.

Grilled Turkey Breast

Cooking Time: 1 hour 30 minutes

Servings: 4

Ingredients:

- 1 whole turkey breast (about 3 pounds)

- Salt and pepper to taste

Instructions:

1. Preheat the grill to medium-high heat.

2. Season the turkey breast with salt and pepper on all sides.

3. Place the turkey breast on the grill and cook for about 1 hour to 1 hour 30 minutes, turning occasionally, or until the internal temperature reaches 165°F (75°C).

4. Remove from the grill and let it rest for 10-15 minutes before slicing.

5. Serve hot.

Nutritional Information: 200 calories, 40g protein, 0g carbohydrates, 0g fiber, 5g fat

Helpful Tip: Brine the turkey breast before grilling for extra moisture and flavor.

Pork Belly Slices

Cooking Time: 45 minutes

Servings: 4

Ingredients:

- 1 lb pork belly, sliced

- Salt and pepper to taste

Instructions:

1. Preheat the oven to 375°F (190°C).

2. Season the pork belly slices with salt and pepper on both sides.

3. Place the pork belly slices on a baking sheet lined with parchment paper.

4. Bake in the preheated oven for about 40-45 minutes, flipping halfway through, or until crispy and cooked through.

5. Remove from the oven and let them rest for a few minutes before serving.

6. Serve hot.

Nutritional Information: 300 calories, 20g protein, 0g carbohydrates, 0g fiber, 25g fat

Helpful Tip: For extra crispiness, broil the pork belly slices for a few minutes at the end of cooking.

Grilled Chicken Wings

Cooking Time: 30 minutes

Servings: 4

Ingredients:

- 2 lbs chicken wings

- Salt and pepper to taste

Instructions:

1. Preheat the grill to medium-high heat.

2. Season the chicken wings with salt and pepper.

3. Place the wings on the grill and cook for about 15-20 minutes, turning occasionally, until they are cooked through and crispy.

4. Remove from the grill and let them rest for a few minutes before serving.

5. Serve hot.

Nutritional Information: 250 calories, 20g protein, 0g carbohydrates, 0g fiber, 15g fat

Helpful Tip: Serve with your favorite dipping sauce or dry rub for extra flavor.

Pork Loin Roast

Cooking Time: 1 hour 30 minutes

Servings: 6

Ingredients:

- 2 lbs pork loin roast

- Salt and pepper to taste

Instructions:

1. Preheat the oven to 375°F (190°C).

2. Season the pork loin roast with salt and pepper on all sides.

3. Place the roast in a roasting pan.

4. Roast in the preheated oven for about 1 hour and 15 minutes to 1 hour and 30 minutes, or until the internal temperature reaches 145°F (63°C).

5. Remove from the oven and let it rest for 10-15 minutes before slicing.

6. Serve hot.

Nutritional Information: 300 calories, 40g protein, 0g carbohydrates, 0g fiber, 15g fat

Helpful Tip: For extra flavor, rub the pork loin roast with herbs and spices before roasting.

Grilled Pork Sausages

Cooking Time: 20 minutes

Servings: 4

Ingredients:

- 4 pork sausages

- Salt and pepper to taste

Instructions:

1. Preheat the grill to medium-high heat.

2. Prick the sausages with a fork in a few places to prevent them from bursting.

3. Place the sausages on the grill and cook for about 10 minutes, turning occasionally, until they are cooked through and browned.

4. Remove from the grill and let them rest for a few minutes before serving.

5. Serve hot.

Nutritional Information: 300 calories, 15g protein, 0g carbohydrates, 0g fiber, 25g fat

Helpful Tip: Serve with mustard or sauerkraut for added flavor.

Baked Chicken Drumsticks

Cooking Time: 45 minutes

Servings: 4

Ingredients:

- 8 chicken drumsticks

- Salt and pepper to taste

Instructions:

1. Preheat the oven to 400°F (200°C).

2. Season the chicken drumsticks with salt and pepper.

3. Place the drumsticks on a baking sheet lined with parchment paper.

4. Bake in the preheated oven for about 40-45 minutes, or until the chicken is cooked through and the skin is crispy.

5. Remove from the oven and let them rest for a few minutes before serving.

6. Serve hot.

Nutritional Information: 250 calories, 25g protein, 0g carbohydrates, 0g fiber, 15g fat

Helpful Tip: For extra flavor, brush the drumsticks with your favorite sauce before baking.

Pork Ribeye Steak

Cooking Time: 15 minutes

Servings: 2

Ingredients:

- 2 Pork ribeye steaks (8 oz each)

- Salt and pepper to taste

Instructions:

1. Preheat a skillet over medium-high heat.

2. Season the pork ribeye steaks with salt and pepper on both sides.

3. Place the steaks in the skillet and cook for about 6-8 minutes on each side, or until they reach an internal temperature of 145°F (63°C).

4. Remove from the skillet and let them rest for a few minutes before serving.

5. Serve hot.

Nutritional Information: 400 calories, 40g protein, 0g carbohydrates, 0g fiber, 25g fat

Helpful Tip: Let the steaks rest after cooking to allow the juices to redistribute and keep the meat tender.

Grilled Turkey Burgers

Cooking Time: 15 minutes

Servings: 4

Ingredients:

- 1 lb ground turkey

- Salt and pepper to taste

Instructions:

1. Preheat the grill to medium-high heat.

2. Season the ground turkey with salt and pepper and form into 4 equal-sized patties.

3. Place the turkey burgers on the grill and cook for about 6-8 minutes on each side, or until they reach an internal temperature of 165°F (75°C).

4. Remove from the grill and let them rest for a few minutes before serving.

5. Serve hot.

Nutritional Information: 250 calories, 30g protein, 0g carbohydrates, 0g fiber, 15g fat

Helpful Tip: Serve the turkey burgers with lettuce wraps or on a bed of greens for a low-carb option.

Chapter 7
Seafood Recipes

Grilled Salmon

Cooking Time: 10 minutes

Servings: 2

Ingredients:

- 2 Salmon fillets (6 oz each)

Instructions:

1. Preheat the grill to medium-high heat.

2. Season the salmon fillets with salt and pepper on both sides.

3. Place the fillets on the grill, skin side down, and cook for about 4-5 minutes.

4. Carefully flip the fillets and cook for another 3-4 minutes, or until they reach an internal temperature of 145°F (63°C).

5. Remove from the grill and let them rest for a few minutes before serving.

6. Serve hot.

Nutritional Information: 350 calories, 40g protein, 0g carbohydrates, 0g fiber, 20g fat

Helpful Tip: For extra flavor, brush the salmon fillets with melted butter or olive oil before grilling.

Pan-Seared Scallops

Cooking Time: 5 minutes

Servings: 2

Ingredients:

- 8 large Scallops

- Salt and pepper to taste

- 2 tablespoons butter or cooking fat of choice

Instructions:

1. Heat a skillet over medium-high heat and add butter or cooking fat.

2. Pat the scallops dry with paper towels and season with salt and pepper on both sides.

3. Once the skillet is hot, add the scallops in a single layer, making sure not to overcrowd the pan.

4. Cook for about 2-3 minutes on each side, or until they are golden brown and opaque in the center.

5. Remove from the skillet and let them rest for a minute before serving.

6. Serve hot.

Nutritional Information: 200 calories, 20g protein, 0g carbohydrates, 0g fiber, 15g fat

Helpful Tip: Make sure the scallops are dry before searing to achieve a nice, caramelized crust.

Broiled Lobster Tails

Cooking Time: 10 minutes

Servings: 2

Ingredients:

- 2 Lobster tails
- 2 tablespoons butter, melted
- Lemon wedges for serving

Instructions:

1. Preheat the broiler on high.
2. Use kitchen shears to cut the top of the lobster shell lengthwise, exposing the meat.
3. Gently pull the lobster meat upward through the cut shell, resting it on top.
4. Season the lobster meat with salt and pepper.
5. Place the lobster tails on a baking sheet lined with aluminum foil.
6. Brush the lobster meat with melted butter.
7. Broil the lobster tails for about 8-10 minutes, or until the meat is opaque and slightly browned.
8. Remove from the oven and let them rest for a minute before serving.
9. Serve hot with lemon wedges.

Nutritional Information: 250 calories, 30g protein, 0g carbohydrates, 0g fiber, 15g fat

Helpful Tip: Avoid overcooking the lobster tails to prevent the meat from becoming tough and rubbery.

Grilled Shrimp Skewers

Cooking Time: 6 minutes

Servings: 2

Ingredients:

- 12 large Shrimp, peeled and deveined

- Salt and pepper to taste

- Wooden or metal skewers

Instructions:

1. Preheat the grill to medium-high heat.

2. Season the shrimp with salt and pepper.

3. Thread the shrimp onto skewers, leaving a little space between each one.

4. Place the skewers on the grill and cook for about 2-3 minutes on each side, or until the shrimp are pink and opaque.

5. Remove from the grill and let them rest for a minute before serving.

6. Serve hot.

Nutritional Information: 150 calories, 25g protein, 0g carbohydrates, 0g fiber, 5g fat

Helpful Tip: Soak wooden skewers in water for at least 30 minutes before grilling to prevent them from burning.

Pan-Fried Cod Fillets

Cooking Time: 8 minutes

Servings: 2

Ingredients:

- 2 Cod fillets (6 oz each)

- Salt and pepper to taste

- 2 tablespoons butter or cooking fat of choice

Instructions:

1. Heat a skillet over medium-high heat and add butter or cooking fat.

2. Season the cod fillets with salt and pepper on both sides.

3. Once the skillet is hot, add the cod fillets.

4. Cook for about 3-4 minutes on each side, or until they are golden brown and easily flake with a fork.

5. Remove from the skillet and let them rest for a minute before serving.

6. Serve hot.

Nutritional Information: 200 calories, 30g protein, 0g carbohydrates, 0g fiber, 10g fat

Helpful Tip: For added flavor, sprinkle the cod fillets with lemon juice or your favorite seasoning before cooking.

Broiled Swordfish Steaks

Cooking Time: 12 minutes

Servings: 2

Ingredients:

- 2 Swordfish steaks (6 oz each)

- Salt and pepper to taste

- 2 tablespoons olive oil

- Lemon wedges for serving

Instructions:

1. Preheat the broiler on high.

2. Season the swordfish steaks with salt and pepper on both sides.

3. Place the steaks on a baking sheet lined with aluminum foil.

4. Drizzle olive oil over the swordfish steaks.

5. Broil the steaks for about 6 minutes on each side, or until they are cooked through and slightly browned.

6. Remove from the oven and let them rest for a minute before serving.

7. Serve hot with lemon wedges.

Nutritional Information: 300 calories, 40g protein, 0g carbohydrates, 0g fiber, 15g fat

Helpful Tip: Watch the swordfish closely while broiling to prevent overcooking.

Baked Halibut Fillets

Cooking Time: 15 minutes

Servings: 2

Ingredients:

- 2 Halibut fillets (6 oz each)

- 2 tablespoons butter, melted

- 2 cloves garlic, minced

Instructions:

1. Preheat the oven to 400°F (200°C).
2. Season the halibut fillets with salt and pepper on both sides.
3. Place the fillets in a baking dish.
4. In a small bowl, mix together melted butter and minced garlic.
5. Pour the butter mixture over the halibut fillets.
6. Bake in the preheated oven for about 12-15 minutes, or until the fish is opaque and flakes easily with a fork.
7. Remove from the oven and let them rest for a minute before serving.
8. Serve hot.

Nutritional Information: 250 calories, 35g protein, 0g carbohydrates, 0g fiber, 12g fat

Helpful Tip: Garnish with chopped parsley or dill before serving for a fresh touch.

Grilled Tuna Steaks

Cooking Time: 8 minutes

Servings: 2

Ingredients:

- 2 Tuna steaks (6 oz each)

- Salt and pepper to taste

- 1 tablespoon olive oil

- 1 teaspoon soy sauce (optional)

Instructions:

1. Preheat the grill to medium-high heat.

2. Season the tuna steaks with salt and pepper on both sides.

3. Drizzle olive oil over the tuna steaks and rub to coat.

4. Optionally, brush the steaks with soy sauce for added flavor.

5. Place the steaks on the grill and cook for about 3-4 minutes on each side for medium-rare, or adjust cooking time according to desired doneness.

6. Remove from the grill and let them rest for a minute before serving.

7. Serve hot.

Nutritional Information: 300 calories, 40g protein, 0g carbohydrates, 0g fiber, 15g fat

Helpful Tip: Avoid overcooking the tuna steaks to prevent them from becoming dry.

Pan-Seared Crab Cakes

Cooking Time: 10 minutes

Servings: 2

Ingredients:

- 1 cup crab meat
- 1 egg
- 2 tablespoons mayonnaise
- 1 teaspoon Dijon mustard
- 2 tablespoons almond flour
- 2 tablespoons butter or cooking fat of choice

Instructions:

1. In a bowl, combine crab meat, egg, mayonnaise, Dijon mustard, salt, pepper, and almond flour. Mix until well combined.

2. Form the mixture into patties.

3. Heat a skillet over medium-high heat and add butter or cooking fat.

4. Once the skillet is hot, add the crab cakes.

5. Cook for about 4-5 minutes on each side, or until they are golden brown and heated through.

6. Remove from the skillet and let them rest for a minute before serving.

7. Serve hot.

Nutritional Information: 250 calories, 20g protein, 1g carbohydrates, 0g fiber, 18g fat

Helpful Tip: Use lump crab meat for the best texture and flavor in crab cakes.

Broiled Mussels

Cooking Time: 8 minutes

Servings: 2

Ingredients:

- 16 Mussels, cleaned and debearded

- 2 tablespoons butter, melted

- 2 cloves garlic, minced

- 2 tablespoons chopped parsley

Instructions:

1. Preheat the broiler on high.

2. In a bowl, mix together melted butter, minced garlic, chopped parsley, salt, and pepper.

3. Arrange the mussels on a baking sheet lined with aluminum foil.

4. Spoon the butter mixture over the mussels.

5. Broil the mussels for about 4 minutes, or until they open and the edges begin to crisp.

6. Remove from the oven and let them rest for a minute before serving.

7. Serve hot.

Nutritional Information: 150 calories, 10g protein, 2g carbohydrates, 0g fiber, 10g fat

Helpful Tip: Discard any mussels that do not open during cooking.

Grilled Sardines

Cooking Time: 8 minutes

Servings: 2

Ingredients:

- 6 whole Sardines, cleaned and gutted

- Salt and pepper to taste

- Olive oil for brushing

Instructions:

1. Preheat the grill to medium-high heat.

2. Season the sardines with salt and pepper.

3. Brush the sardines lightly with olive oil.

4. Place the sardines on the grill and cook for about 3-4 minutes on each side, or until they are cooked through and slightly charred.

5. Remove from the grill and let them rest for a minute before serving.

6. Serve hot.

Nutritional Information: 200 calories, 20g protein, 0g carbohydrates, 0g fiber, 12g fat

Helpful Tip: Serve the grilled sardines with lemon wedges and a sprinkle of chopped fresh herbs for added flavor.

Pan-Fried Anchovy Fillets

Cooking Time: 5 minutes

Servings: 2

Ingredients:

- 8 Anchovy fillets, cleaned and deboned

- Salt and pepper to taste

- 2 tablespoons butter or cooking fat of choice

Instructions:

1. Heat a skillet over medium-high heat and add butter or cooking fat.

2. Season the anchovy fillets with salt and pepper.

3. Once the skillet is hot, add the anchovy fillets.

4. Cook for about 1-2 minutes on each side, or until they are golden brown and crispy.

5. Remove from the skillet and let them rest for a minute before serving.

6. Serve hot.

Nutritional Information: 150 calories, 15g protein, 0g carbohydrates, 0g fiber, 10g fat

Helpful Tip: Anchovy fillets cook very quickly, so be careful not to overcook them to prevent them from becoming dry.

Chapter 8
Desserts & Snacks

Bacon-Wrapped Dates

Cooking Time: 20 minutes

Servings: 4

Ingredients:

- 8 Medjool dates, pitted

- 4 slices bacon, cut in half crosswise

Instructions:

1. Preheat the oven to 375°F (190°C).

2. Stuff each date with a piece of bacon.

3. Wrap the bacon around the date and secure with a toothpick.

4. Place the bacon-wrapped dates on a baking sheet lined with parchment paper.

5. Bake in the preheated oven for about 15-20 minutes, or until the bacon is crispy.

6. Remove from the oven and let them cool slightly before serving.

7. Serve warm.

Nutritional Information: 150 calories, 3g protein, 20g carbohydrates, 2g fiber, 7g fat

Helpful Tip: Choose thick-cut bacon for better wrapping and flavor.

Cheese Crisps

Cooking Time: 10 minutes

Servings: 4

Ingredients:

- 1 cup shredded cheddar cheese

Instructions:

1. Preheat the oven to 400°F (200°C).

2. Line a baking sheet with parchment paper.

3. Place small piles of shredded cheddar cheese on the prepared baking sheet, leaving space between each pile.

4. Flatten each pile slightly with your fingers.

5. Bake in the preheated oven for about 6-8 minutes, or until the edges are golden brown and crispy.

6. Remove from the oven and let them cool completely before serving.

7. Serve as crispy cheese snacks.

Nutritional Information: 100 calories, 6g protein, 1g carbohydrates, 0g fiber, 8g fat

Helpful Tip: Experiment with different types of cheese for variety.

Beef Jerky

Cooking Time: 4-6 hours

Servings: 4

Ingredients:

- 1 lb beef sirloin or flank steak, thinly sliced against the grain

- Salt and pepper to taste

- Optional seasonings: garlic powder, onion powder, smoked paprika

Instructions:

1. Preheat the oven to 175°F (80°C) or the lowest setting.

2. Season the thinly sliced beef with salt, pepper, and any optional seasonings of your choice.

3. Arrange the beef slices on a baking sheet lined with parchment paper, making sure they don't overlap.

4. Place the baking sheet in the oven and bake for 4-6 hours, or until the beef is dried and chewy.

5. Remove from the oven and let the beef jerky cool completely before serving.

6. Store in an airtight container for up to 2 weeks.

Nutritional Information: 120 calories, 20g protein, 0g carbohydrates, 0g fiber, 4g fat

Helpful Tip: Marinate the beef slices in your favorite low-carb marinade before drying for extra flavor.

Pepperoni Chips

Cooking Time: 10 minutes

Servings: 4

Ingredients:

- 20 slices pepperoni

Instructions:

1. Preheat the oven to 400°F (200°C).

2. Line a baking sheet with parchment paper.

3. Place the pepperoni slices in a single layer on the prepared baking sheet.

4. Bake in the preheated oven for about 8-10 minutes, or until the pepperoni slices are crispy.

5. Remove from the oven and let them cool slightly before serving.

6. Serve as crispy pepperoni chips.

Nutritional Information: 120 calories, 5g protein, 1g carbohydrates, 0g fiber, 10g fat

Helpful Tip: Blot excess grease from the pepperoni slices with paper towels after baking for crispier chips.

Devilled Eggs

Cooking Time: 15 minutes

Servings: 4

Ingredients:

- 4 large eggs
- 2 tablespoons mayonnaise
- 1 teaspoon mustard
- Paprika for garnish (optional)

Instructions:

1. Place the eggs in a saucepan and cover with water.
2. Bring the water to a boil, then reduce the heat to low and simmer for 10 minutes.
3. Remove the eggs from the water and let them cool completely.
4. Peel the eggs and cut them in half lengthwise. Remove the yolks and place them in a bowl.
5. Mash the egg yolks with mayonnaise, mustard, salt, and pepper until smooth.
6. Spoon or pipe the yolk mixture back into the egg white halves.
7. Garnish with paprika if desired.
8. Serve chilled.

Nutritional Information: 150 calories, 8g protein, 1g carbohydrates, 0g fiber, 12g fat

Helpful Tip: For easier peeling, use eggs that are at least a week old.

Prosciutto-Wrapped Mozzarella Sticks

Cooking Time: 10 minutes

Servings: 4

Ingredients:

- 8 mozzarella cheese sticks

- 8 slices prosciutto

Instructions:

1. Preheat the oven to 400°F (200°C).

2. Wrap each mozzarella cheese stick with a slice of prosciutto.

3. Place the wrapped cheese sticks on a baking sheet lined with parchment paper.

4. Bake in the preheated oven for about 8-10 minutes, or until the prosciutto is crispy and the cheese is melted.

5. Remove from the oven and let them cool slightly before serving.

6. Serve warm.

Nutritional Information: 200 calories, 16g protein, 1g carbohydrates, 0g fiber, 15g fat

Helpful Tip: Serve with marinara sauce for dipping if desired.

Chicken Liver Pâté

Cooking Time: 20 minutes
Servings: 4

Ingredients:

- 1 lb chicken livers, trimmed
- 1 small onion, finely chopped
- 2 cloves garlic, minced
- Optional: herbs and spices of your choice

Instructions:

1. In a skillet, melt 2 tablespoons of butter over medium heat.
2. Add the chopped onion and minced garlic to the skillet and cook until softened, about 3-4 minutes.
3. Add the chicken livers to the skillet and cook until browned on the outside but still slightly pink on the inside, about 3-4 minutes per side.
4. Transfer the cooked chicken livers, onions, and garlic to a food processor.
5. Add the remaining butter and any optional herbs and spices to the food processor.
6. Process until smooth and creamy.
7. Season with salt and pepper to taste.
8. Transfer the pâté to a serving dish or storage container.
9. Cover and refrigerate for at least 2 hours before serving.
10. Serve chilled.

Nutritional Information: 250 calories, 20g protein, 2g carbohydrates, 0g fiber, 18g fat

Beef Bone Broth

Cooking Time: 12-24 hours

Servings: Varies

Ingredients:

- 4 lbs beef bones (marrow bones, knuckle bones, or a mixture)

- Optional: salt, pepper, herbs, and spices of your choice

Instructions:

1. Preheat the oven to 400°F (200°C).
2. Place the beef bones on a baking sheet and roast in the preheated oven for about 30 minutes, or until browned.
3. Transfer the roasted bones to a large stockpot or slow cooker.
4. Cover the bones with water by about 2 inches.
5. Bring the water to a gentle boil, then reduce the heat to low and simmer for 12-24 hours, skimming any foam that rises to the surface.
6. If using a slow cooker, set it to low and let it simmer for 12-24 hours.
7. Add salt, pepper, herbs, and spices to taste during the last hour of cooking.
8. Once the broth is done, strain it through a fine-mesh sieve or cheesecloth to remove any solids.
9. Let the broth cool, then transfer it to storage containers.
10. Refrigerate for up to 5 days or freeze for longer storage.
11. Reheat before serving.

Nutritional Information: Varies depending on ingredients

Helpful Tip: Enjoy a warm cup of beef bone broth as a comforting and nourishing snack.

Pork Rinds

Cooking Time: 20 minutes

Servings: 4

Ingredients:

- 1 lb pork skin, cut into strips
- Salt to taste

Instructions:

1. Preheat the oven to 375°F (190°C).
2. Place the pork skin strips on a baking sheet lined with parchment paper.
3. Sprinkle salt evenly over the pork skin strips.
4. Bake in the preheated oven for about 15-20 minutes, or until the pork skin is crispy and golden brown.
5. Remove from the oven and let them cool slightly before serving.
6. Serve as crunchy pork rinds.

Nutritional Information: 180 calories, 10g protein, 0g carbohydrates, 0g fiber, 15g fat

Helpful Tip: Experiment with different seasonings like garlic powder or chili powder for extra flavor.

Salami Chips

Cooking Time: 10 minutes

Servings: 4

Ingredients:

- 20 slices salami

Instructions:

1. Preheat the oven to 400°F (200°C).

2. Line a baking sheet with parchment paper.

3. Place the salami slices in a single layer on the prepared baking sheet.

4. Bake in the preheated oven for about 8-10 minutes, or until the salami slices are crispy.

5. Remove from the oven and let them cool slightly before serving.

6. Serve as crispy salami chips.

Nutritional Information: 160 calories, 8g protein, 1g carbohydrates, 0g fiber, 12g fat

Helpful Tip: Blot excess grease from the salami slices with paper towels after baking for crispier chips.

Chapter 7
Nose to Tail Recipes

Beef Heart Stew

Cooking Time: 2 hours 30 minutes

Servings: 6

Ingredients:

- 1 beef heart, cleaned and chopped into cubes

- 4 cups beef bone broth

- Salt and pepper to taste

Instructions:

1. In a large pot, bring the beef bone broth to a boil.

2. Add the chopped beef heart to the boiling broth.

3. Reduce the heat to low and simmer for about 2 hours, or until the beef heart is tender.

4. Season with salt and pepper to taste.

5. Serve hot as a nourishing stew.

Nutritional Information: 250 calories, 30g protein, 0g carbohydrates, 0g fiber, 15g fat

Helpful Tip: For added flavor, you can add herbs and spices such as thyme or garlic.

Lamb Brain Omelette

Cooking Time: 15 minutes

Servings: 2

Ingredients:

- 4 lamb brains
- 4 eggs
- Salt and pepper to taste
- Butter for frying

Instructions:

1. Rinse the lamb brains under cold water and pat them dry.
2. In a bowl, beat the eggs and season with salt and pepper.
3. Heat butter in a skillet over medium heat.
4. Dip each lamb brain into the beaten eggs, coating it thoroughly.
5. Place the lamb brains in the skillet and cook for about 3-4 minutes on each side, or until golden brown and cooked through.
6. Serve hot as an omelette.

Nutritional Information: 300 calories, 25g protein, 1g carbohydrates, 0g fiber, 20g fat

Helpful Tip: Be gentle when handling lamb brains as they are delicate and can break easily.

Pork Kidney Stir-Fry

Cooking Time: 20 minutes

Servings: 4

Ingredients:

- 2 pork kidneys, cleaned and thinly sliced

- 2 tablespoons butter or cooking fat of choice

- Salt and pepper to taste

Instructions:

1. Heat butter or cooking fat in a skillet over medium-high heat.

2. Add the sliced pork kidneys to the skillet and cook for about 5-7 minutes, or until they are browned.

3. Season with salt and pepper to taste.

4. Serve hot as a flavorful stir-fry.

Nutritional Information: 180 calories, 20g protein, 0g carbohydrates, 0g fiber, 12g fat

Helpful Tip: Soak the pork kidneys in milk for a few hours before cooking to reduce their strong flavor.

Beef Tongue Tacos

Cooking Time: 4 hours 30 minutes

Servings: 4

Ingredients:

- 1 beef tongue
- 1 onion, chopped
- 4 cloves garlic, minced
- 2 cups beef broth
- Lettuce leaves (for serving)
- Salsa (for serving)
- Sour cream (for serving)

Instructions:

1. Place the beef tongue in a slow cooker and add chopped onion, minced garlic, and beef broth.
2. Cook on low heat for about 4 hours, or until the beef tongue is tender.
3. Remove the beef tongue from the slow cooker and let it cool slightly.
4. Peel off the outer layer of skin from the beef tongue and discard.
5. Slice the beef tongue thinly.
6. Serve the sliced beef tongue in lettuce leaves with salsa and sour cream.

Nutritional Information: 300 calories, 25g protein, 2g carbohydrates, 0g fiber, 20g fat

Helpful Tip: Beef tongue is best cooked low and slow to ensure tenderness.

Chicken Feet Broth

Cooking Time: 3 hours

Servings: 6

Ingredients:

- 1 lb chicken feet
- 8 cups water
- Salt to taste

Instructions:

1. Rinse the chicken feet under cold water and place them in a large pot.
2. Cover the chicken feet with water and bring to a boil over high heat.
3. Reduce the heat to low and simmer for about 3 hours, skimming any foam that rises to the surface.
4. Season with salt to taste.
5. Strain the broth through a fine-mesh sieve.
6. Serve hot as a comforting and nourishing broth.

Nutritional Information: 50 calories, 5g protein, 0g carbohydrates, 0g fiber, 3g fat

Helpful Tip: Chicken feet are rich in collagen, which contributes to the gelatinous texture of the broth when cooked.

Beef Marrow Roast

Cooking Time: 1 hour 30 minutes

Servings: 4

Ingredients:

- 4 beef marrow bones, cut lengthwise

- Salt and pepper to taste

Instructions:

1. Preheat the oven to 375°F (190°C).

2. Place the beef marrow bones on a baking sheet lined with parchment paper.

3. Season with salt and pepper.

4. Roast in the preheated oven for about 1 hour, or until the marrow is soft and begins to bubble.

5. Remove from the oven and let them cool slightly.

6. Serve hot, scooping out the marrow with a spoon.

Nutritional Information: 200 calories, 15g protein, 0g carbohydrates, 0g fiber, 15g fat

Helpful Tip: Serve the roasted beef marrow with crusty bread or enjoy it on its own.

Lamb Sweetbreads with Lemon Butter Sauce

Cooking Time: 30 minutes

Servings: 4

Ingredients:

- 1 lb lamb sweetbreads
- 2 tablespoons butter
- 2 cloves garlic, minced
- Juice of 1 lemon
- 1 tablespoon chopped parsley

Instructions:

1. Rinse the lamb sweetbreads under cold water and pat them dry with paper towels. Remove any excess fat or membrane.
2. Season the sweetbreads with salt and pepper.
3. Heat butter in a skillet over medium-high heat.
4. Add the lamb sweetbreads to the skillet and cook for about 5-7 minutes on each side, or until golden brown and cooked through.
5. Add minced garlic to the skillet and cook for another minute.
6. Pour lemon juice over the sweetbreads and sprinkle with chopped parsley.
7. Serve hot, spooning the lemon butter sauce over the sweetbreads.

Nutritional Information: 250 calories, 20g protein, 1g carbohydrates, 0g fiber, 18g fat

Helpful Tip: Soak the lamb sweetbreads in milk for a few hours before cooking to remove any excess blood and milder their flavor.

Pork Tail Stew

Cooking Time: 3 hours 30 minutes

Servings: 6

Ingredients:

- 2 lbs pork tails, chopped into pieces
- 4 cups beef bone broth
- 1 onion, chopped
- 2 cloves garlic, minced
- Salt and pepper to taste

Instructions:

1. In a large pot, combine pork tails, beef bone broth, chopped onion, and minced garlic.

2. Bring to a boil over high heat, then reduce the heat to low and simmer, covered, for about 3 hours.

3. Season with salt and pepper to taste.

4. Serve hot as a hearty stew.

Nutritional Information: 300 calories, 25g protein, 0g carbohydrates, 0g fiber, 20g fat

Helpful Tip: Pork tails are collagen-rich and become tender and flavorful when slow-cooked in a stew.

Beef Tripe Curry

Cooking Time: 2 hours

Servings: 4

Ingredients:

- 1 lb beef tripe, cleaned and sliced
- 2 tablespoons ghee or cooking fat of choice
- 1 onion, finely chopped
- 2 cloves garlic, minced
- 1 tablespoon ginger, minced
- 2 tablespoons curry powder
- 1 cup coconut milk

Instructions:

1. In a large pot, heat ghee over medium heat. Add chopped onion, minced garlic, and minced ginger. Sauté until fragrant.
2. Add sliced beef tripe to the pot and cook until browned.
3. Stir in curry powder and cook for another minute.
4. Pour in coconut milk and bring to a simmer.
5. Reduce heat to low, cover, and simmer for about 1.5 to 2 hours, or until the tripe is tender. Season with salt and pepper to taste.
6. Serve hot with cauliflower rice or enjoy on its own.

Nutritional Information: 280 calories, 20g protein, 5g carbohydrates, 1g fiber, 20g fat

Helpful Tip: Soaking the beef tripe in water with a splash of vinegar for a few hours before cooking can help remove any residual smell and tenderize the tripe.

Lamb Testicles Sautéed with Garlic and Herbs

Cooking Time: 15 minutes

Servings: 4

Ingredients:

- 1 lb lamb testicles
- 2 tablespoons olive oil
- 3 cloves garlic, minced
- 1 tablespoon chopped fresh herbs (such as parsley, thyme, or rosemary)

Instructions:

1. Blanch the lamb testicles in boiling water for about 2-3 minutes. Drain and rinse under cold water.
2. Peel off the tough outer membrane from the lamb testicles and discard.
3. Slice the lamb testicles into thin rounds.
4. Heat olive oil in a skillet over medium-high heat.
5. Add minced garlic to the skillet and sauté until fragrant.
6. Add sliced lamb testicles to the skillet and cook for about 5-7 minutes, or until browned and cooked through.
7. Stir in chopped fresh herbs and season with salt and pepper to taste.
8. Serve hot as a flavorful and nutritious dish.

Nutritional Information: 220 calories, 25g protein, 1g carbohydrates, 0g fiber, 12g fat

Helpful Tip: Lamb testicles are delicate and cook quickly, so be careful not to overcook them to maintain their tenderness.

CONCLUSION

As we reach the culmination of this culinary journey, I am filled with gratitude for the opportunity to share in your pursuit of vitality and well-being. "Carnivore Diet Cookbook for Seniors" has been crafted with love and dedication, with the hope of inspiring transformation and joy in your life.

As you explore the recipes within these pages, may you discover the profound nourishment that real, wholesome foods can offer. From savory steaks to comforting stews, each dish is a testament to the power of nutrition to rejuvenate the body and uplift the spirit.

But our journey does not end here. Your feedback is invaluable in our mission to continually improve and evolve. I invite you to share your thoughts, experiences, and suggestions – your voice is instrumental in shaping future editions and ensuring that " Carnivore Diet Cookbook for Seniors " continues to inspire and empower others on their path to wellness.

If you've found this cookbook to be a source of joy and nourishment, I humbly ask for your support in spreading the word. Your positive reviews and recommendations can help guide others toward a life filled with vitality and abundance.

Thank you for entrusting me with a part of your journey. May your days be filled with laughter, love, and the simple joys of savouring life's most precious moments.

BONUS 1
30 Day Meal Plan

Day	Breakfast	Lunch	Dinner
1	Scrambled Eggs	Grilled Chicken Thighs	Beef Burger with Cheese
2	Bacon and Sausage	Beef Liver Pâté	Pan-Seared Salmon
3	Beef Bone Broth	Pork Rinds	Lamb Chops
4	Omelette with Ham	Chicken Caesar Salad	Ribeye Steak
5	Pork Belly Slices	Beef Heart Stew	Grilled Shrimp
6	Beef Sausage Links	Pork Ribs	Lamb Shoulder Chops
7	Breakfast Sausage Patties	Beef Marrow Roast	Chicken Drumsticks
8	Smoked Salmon	Beef Tongue Tacos	Bacon-Wrapped Filet Mignon
9	Beef Jerky	Chicken Liver Pâté	Grilled Pork Chops
10	Beef Short Ribs	Pork Tail Stew	Pan-Seared Duck Breast
11	Ham Steak	Beef Tripe Curry	Grilled Lamb Kabobs
12	Lamb Bacon	Beef Tongue Stew	Seared Tuna Steaks
13	Ribeye Steak and Eggs	Pork Kidney Stir-Fry	Chicken Wings
14	Corned Beef Hash	Beef Brisket	Grilled Turkey Breast

15	Breakfast Burger	Lamb Sweetbreads with Lemon Butter Sauce	Bacon-Wrapped Scallops
16	Chicken Sausage Links	Pork Belly Burnt Ends	Beef Chuck Roast
17	Smoked Ham	Beef Liver and Onions	Grilled Pork Tenderloin
18	Beef Breakfast Patties	Lamb Brain Omelette	Pan-Seared Halibut
19	Canadian Bacon	Pork Loin Chops	Grilled Salmon
20	Beef Kabobs	Beef Tallow Fries	Roast Duck
21	Steak and Eggs	Lamb Curry	Bacon-Wrapped Chicken Thighs
22	Pulled Pork	Beef Heart Salad	Seared Swordfish Steaks
23	Breakfast Sausage Links	Pork Rind Nachos	Grilled Sardines
24	Lamb Sausage Patties	Beef Bone Broth Soup	Pan-Seared Scallops
25	Ham and Cheese Omelette	Pork Loin Roast	Grilled T-bone Steak
26	Bacon and Eggs	Beef Tripe Soup	Broiled Lobster Tails
27	Beef Breakfast Sausage	Pork Liver Pâté	Seared Ahi Tuna
28	Canadian Bacon and Eggs	Lamb Testicles Sautéed	Grilled Mahi Mahi
29	Pork Sausage Patties	Beef Tongue Salad	Pan-Fried Anchovy Fillets
30	Smoked Turkey Legs	Beef Marrow Soup	Grilled Octopus

REVIEW PAGE

Thank you for choosing to embark on this journey with me through the pages of **"CARNIVORE DIET COOKBOOK FOR SENOIRS"** Your decision to invest in my work means the world to me, and I am deeply grateful for your support.

As an author, there's nothing quite as rewarding as knowing that my words have resonated with someone like you. Now that you've experienced the story, I would greatly appreciate your feedback. Your honest review is not only invaluable in helping me grow as a writer but also serves as a source of motivation to continue creating.

Please consider leaving a honest review on my book.

Your support and encouragement mean everything to me. Thank you for being a part of this journey.

BONUS 2
MEAL PLANNER JOURNAL

WEEKLY —

Meal Planner

Week of:

Monday	Tuesday	Wednesday
BREAKFAST	BREAKFAST	BREAKFAST
LUNCH	LUNCH	LUNCH
DINNER	DINNER	DINNER
SNACK	SNACK	SNACK

Thursday	Friday	Saturday
BREAKFAST	BREAKFAST	BREAKFAST
LUNCH	LUNCH	LUNCH
DINNER	DINNER	DINNER
SNACK	SNACK	SNACK

Sunday	NOTES:
BREAKFAST	
LUNCH	
DINNER	
SNACK	

Meal Planner

Week of:

| | Monday | | Tuesday | | Wednesday |

Monday

BREAKFAST

LUNCH

DINNER

SNACK

Tuesday

BREAKFAST

LUNCH

DINNER

SNACK

Wednesday

BREAKFAST

LUNCH

DINNER

SNACK

Thursday

BREAKFAST

LUNCH

DINNER

SNACK

Friday

BREAKFAST

LUNCH

DINNER

SNACK

Saturday

BREAKFAST

LUNCH

DINNER

SNACK

Sunday

BREAKFAST

LUNCH

DINNER

SNACK

NOTES:

Meal Planner

Week of:

	Monday
BREAKFAST	
LUNCH	
DINNER	
SNACK	

	Tuesday
BREAKFAST	
LUNCH	
DINNER	
SNACK	

	Wednesday
BREAKFAST	
LUNCH	
DINNER	
SNACK	

	Thursday
BREAKFAST	
LUNCH	
DINNER	
SNACK	

	Friday
BREAKFAST	
LUNCH	
DINNER	
SNACK	

	Saturday
BREAKFAST	
LUNCH	
DINNER	
SNACK	

	Sunday
BREAKFAST	
LUNCH	
DINNER	
SNACK	

NOTES:

Meal Planner

Week of:

Monday	Tuesday	Wednesday
BREAKFAST	BREAKFAST	BREAKFAST
LUNCH	LUNCH	LUNCH
DINNER	DINNER	DINNER
SNACK	SNACK	SNACK

Thursday	Friday	Saturday
BREAKFAST	BREAKFAST	BREAKFAST
LUNCH	LUNCH	LUNCH
DINNER	DINNER	DINNER
SNACK	SNACK	SNACK

Sunday	NOTES:
BREAKFAST	
LUNCH	
DINNER	
SNACK	

Meal Planner

Week of:

Monday

BREAKFAST

LUNCH

DINNER

SNACK

Tuesday

BREAKFAST

LUNCH

DINNER

SNACK

Wednesday

BREAKFAST

LUNCH

DINNER

SNACK

Thursday

BREAKFAST

LUNCH

DINNER

SNACK

Friday

BREAKFAST

LUNCH

DINNER

SNACK

Saturday

BREAKFAST

LUNCH

DINNER

SNACK

Sunday

BREAKFAST

LUNCH

DINNER

SNACK

NOTES:

Meal Planner

Week of:

Monday

BREAKFAST

LUNCH

DINNER

SNACK

Tuesday

BREAKFAST

LUNCH

DINNER

SNACK

Wednesday

BREAKFAST

LUNCH

DINNER

SNACK

Thursday

BREAKFAST

LUNCH

DINNER

SNACK

Friday

BREAKFAST

LUNCH

DINNER

SNACK

Saturday

BREAKFAST

LUNCH

DINNER

SNACK

Sunday

BREAKFAST

LUNCH

DINNER

SNACK

NOTES:

Meal Planner

Week of:

Monday	Tuesday	Wednesday
BREAKFAST	BREAKFAST	BREAKFAST
LUNCH	LUNCH	LUNCH
DINNER	DINNER	DINNER
SNACK	SNACK	SNACK

Thursday	Friday	Saturday
BREAKFAST	BREAKFAST	BREAKFAST
LUNCH	LUNCH	LUNCH
DINNER	DINNER	DINNER
SNACK	SNACK	SNACK

Sunday	NOTES:
BREAKFAST	
LUNCH	
DINNER	
SNACK	

Meal Planner

Week of:

Monday

BREAKFAST

LUNCH

DINNER

SNACK

Tuesday

BREAKFAST

LUNCH

DINNER

SNACK

Wednesday

BREAKFAST

LUNCH

DINNER

SNACK

Thursday

BREAKFAST

LUNCH

DINNER

SNACK

Friday

BREAKFAST

LUNCH

DINNER

SNACK

Saturday

BREAKFAST

LUNCH

DINNER

SNACK

Sunday

BREAKFAST

LUNCH

DINNER

SNACK

NOTES:

Meal Planner

Week of:

Monday

BREAKFAST

LUNCH

DINNER

SNACK

Tuesday

BREAKFAST

LUNCH

DINNER

SNACK

Wednesday

BREAKFAST

LUNCH

DINNER

SNACK

Thursday

BREAKFAST

LUNCH

DINNER

SNACK

Friday

BREAKFAST

LUNCH

DINNER

SNACK

Saturday

BREAKFAST

LUNCH

DINNER

SNACK

Sunday

BREAKFAST

LUNCH

DINNER

SNACK

NOTES:

Meal Planner

Week of:

Monday	**Tuesday**	**Wednesday**
BREAKFAST	BREAKFAST	BREAKFAST
LUNCH	LUNCH	LUNCH
DINNER	DINNER	DINNER
SNACK	SNACK	SNACK
Thursday	**Friday**	**Saturday**
BREAKFAST	BREAKFAST	BREAKFAST
LUNCH	LUNCH	LUNCH
DINNER	DINNER	DINNER
SNACK	SNACK	SNACK

Sunday

BREAKFAST

LUNCH

DINNER

SNACK

NOTES:

www.ingramcontent.com/pod-product-compliance
Lightning Source LLC
Chambersburg PA
CBHW081215260726
48653CB00010BA/3661